LONG TERM CARE

LONG TERM CARE

An Annotated Bibliography

Compiled by
THEODORE H. KOFF
and
KRISTINE M. BURSAC

Bibliographies and Indexes in Gerontology, Number 25
Erdman B. Palmore, *Series Adviser*

Greenwood Press
Westport, Connecticut • London

Library of Congress Cataloging-in-Publication Data

Long term care : an annotated bibliography / compiled by Theodore H.
Koff and Kristine M. Bursac.
        p.   cm.—(Bibliographies and indexes in gerontology, ISSN
0743–7560 ; no. 25)
        Includes index.
        ISBN 0–313–28583–7 (acid-free paper)
        1. Aged—Long-term care—Bibliography.   2. Chronically ill—Long-
term care—Bibliography.   I. Koff, Theodore H.   II. Bursac, Kristine M.
III. Series.
Z7164.04L55   1995
[HV1451]
016.3621′ 6—dc20   94–39768

British Library Cataloguing in Publication Data is available.

Library of Congress Catalog Card Number: 94–39768
ISBN: 0–313–28583–7
ISSN: 0743–7560

First published in 1995

Greenwood Press, 88 Post Road West, Westport, CT 06881
An imprint of Greenwood Publishing Group, Inc.

Printed in the United States of America

The paper used in this book complies with the
Permanent Paper Standard issued by the National
Information Standards Organization (Z39.48–1984).

10 9 8 7 6 5 4 3 2 1

Contents

Series Foreword

The annotated bibliographies in this series provide answers to the fundamental question, "What is known?" Their purpose is simple, yet profound: to provide comprehensive reviews and references for the work done in various fields of gerontology. They are based on the fact that it is no longer possible for anyone to comprehend the vast body of research and writing in even one sub-specialty without years of work.

This fact has become true only in recent years. When I was an undergraduate (Class of '52) I think no one at Duke had even heard of gerontology. Almost no one in the world was identified as a gerontologist. Now there are over 6,000 professional members of the Gerontological Society of America. When I was an undergraduate, there were no courses in gerontology. Now there are thousands of courses offered by most major (and many minor) colleges and universities. When I was an undergraduate, there was only one gerontological journal (the *Journal of Gerontology*, begun in 1945). Now there are over forty professional journals and several dozen books in gerontology published each year.

The reasons for this dramatic growth are well known: the dramatic increase in numbers of aged, the shift from family to public responsibility for the security and care of the elderly, the recognition of aging as a "social problem"; and the growth of science in general. It is less well known that this explosive growth in knowledge has developed the need for new solutions to the old problem of comprehending and "keeping up" with a field of knowledge. The old indexes and library card catalogues have become increasingly inadequate for the job. On-line computer indexes and abstracts are one solution but make no evaluative selections nor organize sources logically as is done here. These annotated bibliographies are also more widely available than on-line computer indexes.

These bibliographies will obviously be useful for students, teachers, and researchers who need to know what research has (or has not) been done in their field. This particular bibliography will also be useful to long term care administrators, physicians, mental health workers, geriatricians, nurses, nurses aides, and clinical social workers. The annotations contain enough information so that the user usually does not have to search out the original articles.

In the past, the "review of literature" has often been haphazard and was rarely comprehensive, because of the large investment of time (and money) that would be required by a truly comprehensive review. Now, using these bibliographies, researchers and others concerned with this topic can be more confident that they are not missing important previous research and other reports; they can be more confident that they are not duplicating past efforts and "reinventing the wheel." It may well become standard and expected practice for researchers to consult such bibliographies, even before they start their research.

The research relevant to long term care has become a large and rapidly growing field, especially in the last decade. This is attested to by the 249 references in this bibliography, and by the wide variety of disciplines represented here. Thus this volume will be useful to teachers, other professionals, and researchers in many different fields.

The author has done an outstanding job of covering the recent literature and organizing it into easily accessible form. Not only are the entries organized into 12 chapters and numerous subsections, but there is an introduction, and a comprehensive subject index and author index.

Thus one can look for relevant material in this volume in several ways: (1) look up a given subject in the subject index; (2) look up a given author in the author index; or (3) turn to the section and sub-section that covers the subject in which you are interested.

Theodore Koff is exceptionally well-qualified to produce this bibliography. He has long been a specialist in this area, has done significant research, and has published several articles and books on long term care.

So it is with great pleasure that we add this bibliography to our series. We believe you will find this volume to be the most useful, comprehensive, and easily accessible reference work in its field. I will appreciate any comments you care to send me.

Erdman B. Palmore

Acknowledgments

Compiling a bibliography with numerous entries requires enormous effort: searching for the resources, reviewing quantities of materials and finding the appropriate way to capture the essence of the meaning of each document in a few sentences.

Major portions of this activity were conducted by Melissa Murray, Ron Shull, Richard Park, and Lynne Tomasa. We are grateful to them for their diligent approach to this responsibility.

The manuscript was prepared by Lana Myers and edited by Barbara Sears. Their work is always of the highest quality.

Also assisting were Rebecca Butler, Kelly Davis, Anne Fletcher, Amy Hamilton, John Schneiter, and Mark Tibbitts. We wish to express our appreciation to all of them.

Theodore H. Koff and Kristine M. Bursac

Introduction

If we were to ask you, as a reader of this bibliography, to define what long term care means to you, we might expect a variety of responses mentioning nursing homes, care of the elderly, care at home, post-hospital care, chronic care, home health, assisted living, family support, Medicare, Medicaid and much more. These diverse replies illustrate the absence of clarity about what we refer to as long term care. Everyone senses that it differs from acute care, but most of us are not sure about the lines of demarcation that separate the two -- if, in fact, they do differ. It is difficult to fit such important issues as wellness, disease prevention and the maintenance of health into the framework of long term care. We often are misled into believing that it is *duration*, long term, that defines the uniqueness of this field of study and service. In fact, it is not the length of time that a service may be offered that is significant but rather that long term care, if it is to be a significant discipline, should be responsive to the unique needs of the client group who require *chronic* care service.

What then is the operative description for what we refer to as long term care? The essential issue is that suitable responses to chronic illness are different from appropriate responses to acute illness. The issue of chronicity implies a long-standing impairment, a disability resulting in some change in life-style, an accommodation to changes in activities of daily living, a problem without cure. Within this framework it is understandable that "long term" has been used as a synonym for chronicity. Yet we would advocate a continued search for cure for chronic illness as well as for understanding that impairments do not always need to result in long-standing disability, that appropriate and timely intervention not only may reduce the duration of impairment but also, most optimistically, may avert the occurrence of chronicity. Wellness, with all of its related activities of diet, emotional supports, exercise and restriction of harmful activities, may assume greater importance in the field of long term care than is implied by focusing on length of time of service. Short term interventions at the appropriate time may, in fact, prevent the need for long term intervention. Nevertheless, it is not suggested that this type of intervention be referred to as short term care.

The critical concepts are making appropriate responses to the needs of persons with chronic illness, preventing chronic illness and conducting the research necessary to minimize adverse experiences with chronic illness.

Although chronic conditions occur most frequently in older persons, chronic care issues are not restricted to them. When chronicity does occur, it oftentimes has major impacts on activities of daily living. Sometimes this may require institutionalization but, for the most part, persons with chronic illness continue to live at home tending to their own needs. Chronic care, therefore, deals with both institutionalization and the provision of home-delivered services. The most significant number of caregivers to older persons living at home with some impositions on their functional capacity are relatives, with a female child, female relative or daughter-in-law usually carrying the greatest burden of caregiving. For this reason, issues of chronic care also must deal with family caregivers, support of family members and augmenting family resources.

Chronic care services are expensive, especially if they are of long duration and require a significant amount of intervention, as is the case for intensive services delivered at home on a recurrent basis or institutionalization. Finances, costs and ways of delivering services that enable people in need to have access to the required services must be addressed, as must the suitable design of institutional buildings, home modification and adaptation to the needs of the residents and accessibility of home and public places. New systems of delivery of service have to be explored to assure that an individual in need of care receives appropriate services, understands the options for services and is assured of retaining personal dignity even when dependent upon others for help.

Chronic care services may sometimes be provided in acute care settings because of the simultaneous presence of an acute illness or a need for specialized services that are available in that setting. When chronic care services are required concurrently with acute care services, priority often is given to the acute illness. Sometimes formal chronic care services are of brief duration, either because they are provided to individuals who are near death and to those whose family caregivers can provide adequate support.

It should by now be clear that it is our contention that long term care is not the best term to use to describe chronic care services. In using the title "Long Term Care Bibliography," we acknowledge that the field of chronic care is currently widely known as long term care, but we ask you to remember that, however you use it, in teaching or writing, you contribute to an enhanced understanding of chronic care services by engaging in a discussion of why "chronic care" describes the broad scope of services it encompasses far better than the more limited "long term care." We therefore propose a preferred definition of chronic care services.

> Chronic care consists of those services designed to provide diagnostic, preventive, therapeutic, rehabilitative, supportive and maintenance services for individuals who have chronic physical and/or mental impairments in a variety of institutional or non-institutional health settings, including the home, with the goal of promoting the optimum of physical, social and psychological functioning (Koff, 1988).

It is our hope that this brief explanation of the way we approach an understanding of chronic care services will describe the broad selection of resource materials represented in this volume. We think that it is critical to appropriate teaching about chronic care to begin with an understanding of the implications of chronic illness for the individual. We like the concept of the trajectory of chronic illness described by Lubkin (1986) that traces the evolution of chronic illness for an individual, showing the interaction with family, community, living arrangements and finances. We believe that chronic care services cannot be understood without anchoring our thoughts on the person who has the chronic problem, because only then can we appreciate the inconvenience, the pain, the separation from friends and community, the intrusion into life style, the uncertainty of prognosis, the need for palliation, the importance of access to services and the financial resources needed to pay for required services (Strauss, 1984).

It is important to understand the complexity of chronic illness in order to appreciate the complexity of the service system needed to respond to the individual and caregivers, to the illness or multiple illnesses, and to the impact of the illness on the individual over some extended period of time. No single or simple approach can respond to the multiplicity of needs. It should be evident that the response must be equal to the need -- that the complicated presentation of chronic health problems requires effective coordination of diverse services as dictated by the needs of the patient and caregivers.

The highest order of service in the field of chronic illness would be to find ways to avoid illness. Next in importance is to provide services that minimize the complications resulting from chronic conditions, followed by ensuring the availability of access to compassionate services to the person with chronic illness and to his or her family members and caregivers. At all levels of intervention, wellness should be the goal. Wellness can be enhanced by quality care, an understanding of the impacts of chronic illness on life style, development of new interventions that minimize the complications of the illness, the availability of services, and access to funds needed to purchase required services.

We hope the references included in this bibliography will serve as guideposts toward gaining an understanding of the complexity and diversity of the issues related to chronic illness and chronic care services.

References

Koff, T. H. New Approaches to Health Care for an Aging Population. San Francisco, CA: Jossey-Bass, 1988.

Lubkin, I. M. Chronic Illness: Impact and Interventions. Boston, MA: Jones and Bartlett, 1986.

Strauss, A. L. et al. Chronic Illness and the Quality of Life. St. Louis, MO: Mosby, 1984.

LONG TERM CARE

1

Past and Future
of Long Term Care

History

1.   Bulletin of the U.S. Bureau of Labor Statistics. (1925).
The Cost of American Almshouses: Distribution of Almshouses
and Political Unit of Organization. Washington, DC: No. 386.

This report summarized the status of almshouses in America as
of 1925. The study examined the extent to which almshouses
were a distinct part of our country's social order during this time
period and to what degree they were a social and economic
problem.

2.   Caplow, T. (1976). A Brief History of Old-Age Institutions
in the United States. Charlottesville, VA: University of Virginia
Center for Program Effectiveness Studies.

This report explores the relationships between historical changes
in the characteristics of nursing care institutions and the social,
demographic and economic attributes of the older adult
population. Topics presented include: 1) the dependent ages in
England and America (1600-1880); 2) attempts at reforming
institutional poor relief (1880-1930); 3) development of privately-

funded charitable institutions specializing in care of the elderly (1800-1930); and 4) historically operative factors influencing institutionalization of the elderly.

3.   Fox, Daniel M.   (1989).   "Policy and Epidemiology: Financing Health Services for the Chronically Ill and Disabled, 1930-90." The Milbank Quarterly, 67, Suppl. 2, Pt. 2.

This article describes the linkages and interactions of interest groups concerned about compulsory and voluntary health insurance, the growing epidemiological pressure of chronic illness, and 60 years of development of health care financing and policy in the United States. It is shown how the cumulative historical experience of epidemiology has shaped the politics of health policy and insights regarding future financing of health services, especially chronic or long term care, are presented.

4.   Katz, Michael B.   (1984).   "Poorhouses and the Origins of the Public Old Age Home."   Milbank Memorial Fund Quarterly/Health and Society, 62(1):110-40.

The American poorhouse exemplified the welfare policy from which the public old age home evolved. This descriptive study examines the transformation of the poorhouse from serving many diverse groups (homeless, poor, children, insane, aged and chronically sick) into public facilities predominantly serving only the aged. Topics include the origins and program goals of early poorhouses, reasons for failure, success in sustaining the work ethic in 19th-century America, population groups served (children and mentally ill) and reforms leading to shifting their care to other locations and a profile of the old age home.

5.   Moroney, R. and N. Kurtz. (1975). The Evolution of Long Term Care Institutions in Long Term Care: A Handbook for Researchers, Planners and Providers. New York, NY: Spectrum.

This book is a historical analysis of nursing care and related institutions in the United States, with a special focus on their changing relationships with other components in the medical care system. A systems approach was used to examine linkages between nursing homes and other health care organizations, and how these relationships changed over time. The authors describe the systems framework used, analyze various historical periods and project future developments.

6.   Rosenberg, Charles E. (1982). "From Almshouse to Hospital: The Shaping of Philadelphia General Hospital." Milbank Memorial Fund Quarterly/Health and Society, 60(1):108-154.

When Philadelphia General Hospital (PGH) was closed in 1977 it was almost 250 years old and in most ways typified older city municipal hospitals which had developed as welfare institutions. This descriptive profile summarizes the transformation of PGH from an almshouse to a municipal hospital. Areas of discussion include: 1) description of the almshouse environment, administration, social structure and patient population; 2) differences between public and private hospitals in 19th century America (conditions, types of cases [mostly chronic or incurable], work force characteristics [inmate labor], etc.); 3) the medicalization and reform of PGH by physicians; 4) development of nurses' training and recruitment outside the hospital; and 5) status of PGH entering the 20th century.

7.   Somers, Anne R. (1982). "Long Term Care for the Elderly and Disabled: A New Health Priority." The New England Journal of Medicine, 307(4):221-226.

This article compares current public policy positions with possible future provisions and financing of long term care. The author discusses the failure of long term care policies in this country and factors associated with the growing need for a comprehensive long term care policy. The essential elements of a two-part proposal for such a policy are presented   These include integration of acute and long term care for the elderly and disabled populations and call for local or community agencies to carry out the actual case management of individual patients. In addition, an alternative proposal, Local Area Management Organizations (LAMOs), is summarized.

8.   Stotsky, Bernard A. (1966). "Nursing Homes: A Review." American Journal of Psychiatry, 123(3):249-258.

This article explores the evolution of the proprietary nursing home since the passage of the Social Security Act of 1935. The author summarizes the impact of the Medical Assistance to the Aged Act (Kerr-Mills, 1964) on the nursing home industry and problems arising from inadequate provision of psychiatric services. A discussion of the reorganization of medical care systems (focusing on rehabilitation and psychiatric therapy) to accommodate the 1967 provisions of Medicare coverage for extended care facilities is presented. The author encourages psychiatrists to make a major commitment to treating older patients and working with staff in extended care facilities.

Future of Aging

9.   Bass, Scott A., Francis G. Caro and Yung-Ping Chen (Eds.). (1993). Achieving a Productive Aging Society. Westport, CT: Auburn House, 312 pages.

This is a collection of essays concerning older people who seek productive, satisfying economic and social roles in society. While viewing older people as valuable and active individuals, the contributors acknowledged that societal attitudes, policies and ideas inhibit many from reaching their full potential. Topics include employment, volunteer work, caregiving, long term care, religious influences, later-life education, and special populations defined by gender, culture and ethnicity.

10.   Coile, Russell C. (1993). "Future Trends, Health Care Reform and the Outlook for Long Term Care." Journal of Long Term Care Administration, 6-10, Fall.

Predictions are made about the future of health care reform and long term care. As HMOs seek lower-cost alternatives to hospitalization, contracting between nursing homes and HMOs will become more common. Long term care providers will no longer operate in isolation. "Care maps" will be assigned to patients as standard procedure. New technology and "care maps" will revolutionize long term care, according to this author.

11.   Fries, James F. (1990). "The Sunny Side of Aging." Journal of the American Medical Association, 263(17):2354-2355.

This editorial provides an optimistic view of the future health and medical care of an aging population in which problems are not insurmountable and solutions are possible. Two optimistic trends are presented: the slowing of increases in life expectancy and the later onset of disability. A proposed research agenda focuses on the investigation of nonfatal chronic diseases from both biomedical and preventive perspectives.

12.   Himes, Christine L. (1992). "Future Caregivers: Projected Family Structures of Older Persons." Journal of Gerontology: Social Sciences, 47(1):S17-26.

Multiple decrement life tables and component projection methods are used to predict family structures of the future older adult population. The procedure is applied to the U.S. population aged 45 and older in 1980 and estimates the population by age, sex, race and marital status for five-year intervals from 1985 until the year 2020. Data analysis focuses on the effects of demographic factors on future family caregiving (labor force participation, geographic location, etc.) and addresses the capacity and willingness of families to provide care.

13.   Kodner, Dennis L. (1993). "Long Term Care 2010: Speculations and Implications." The Journal of Long Term Care Administration, 82-86, Winter.

Demographic changes, medical breakthroughs and a more affluent clientele will change the ways future nursing homes operate. By the year 2010, the author predicts the following: financing by a combination of public and private sources, local access agencies to coordinate care from a single starting point, managed long term care (much like an HMO or On Lok) and a shift toward in-home and community-based services. As a result, the freestanding long term care facility will cease to exist, having become absorbed by large for-profit and nonprofit chains that provide care based on a standardized quality assurance system. These changes will require more professional management and staff as well as increased use of technology. More emphasis will be placed on prevention. Government and private efforts will collaborate to strengthen informal care and develop alternative financing systems, but these changes will require strong political leadership and the willingness of key interest groups to reform the financing system.

14.   Lewin, Marion Ein and Sean Sullivan. (1989). The Care of Tomorrow's Elderly. Washington, DC: American Enterprise Institute for Public Policy Research, 189 pages.

This book addresses future health care needs of an aging population from a multidisciplinary perspective in light of limited resources. Each chapter is an essay by a different author and offers a cultural, social, or economic solution, rather than a medical one.

15.   Schneider, Edward L. and Jack M. Guralnik. (1990). "The Aging of America: Impact on Health Care Costs." Journal of the American Medical Association, 263(17):2335-2340.

The impact of the "oldest-old" on disability benefits, institutionalization, Medicare costs, nursing home costs and specific problems (dementias and hip fractures) and disorders of aging now and in the future are discussed. Data presenting actual and projected statistics in each area are graphically displayed. The authors conclude that the initiation of cost-containment strategies alone will not reduce escalating health care costs, but must be combined with measures to prevent or cure those age-dependent diseases that produce the greatest needs for chronic care.

16.   Suzman, Richard M., David P. Willis and Kenneth G. Manton (Eds.). (1992). The Oldest Old. New York, NY: Oxford University Press, 444 pages.

The oldest-old, those over the age of 85, are the focus of this book. The authors review the literature on long term care needs of this age group. Future demographic trends are discussed, along with the unique characteristics of this population. A clear distinction is made between chronological age and functional capabilities.

17.   U.S. General Accounting Office. (1991). Long Term Care: Projected Needs of the Aging Baby Boom Generation. Report to the Special Committee on Aging, U.S. Senate. Washington, DC: U.S. Government Printing Office, 22 pages.

This report projecting the long term care needs of the baby boom generation in the years 2018-60 when, based on demographics its numbers are expected to peak, also looks at the ability of the population to pay for required services.

2

Institutional Care

Institutionalization

18.　　Bear, Mary. (1990). "Social Networks and Health: Impact on Returning Home After Entry into Residential Care Homes." The Gerontologist, 30(1):30-34.

This article examines the effects of health, functional and cognitive status, the characteristics of the facility and the dimensions of social networks on the likelihood of returning home from a residential care home (RCH). A longitudinal design was used to collect data from 85 RCH residents (from 47 moderate size RCHs) and 75 of their closest acquaintances. Follow-up interviews were conducted six months later. Study results demonstrate that over one-third of subjects had either relocated or died within six months of entering an RCH; residents at a higher level of physical and mental competence were more likely to return home; and the stronger the social support network at time of entry to an RCH, the less likely it was that the older person would return home.

19.   Bennett, Ruth G. (1963). "The Meaning of Institutional Life." The Gerontologist, 3:117-125.

In this classic essay, the author briefly examines the meaning of institutionalization of the aged from four perspectives: its meaning for society, its sociological meaning, its meaning for professional and administrative staff, and its meaning for residents. Her discussions of the second of these meanings, in which she applies the sociological concept of "total institution" to institutions for the aged and suggests criteria for determining the degree of totality of an institution, has probably been the most influential of the many insights that the article contains.

20.   Braun, Kathryn L., Charles L. Rose and Michael D. Finch. (1991). "Patient Characteristics and Outcomes in Institutional and Community Long Term Care." The Gerontologist, 31(5):648-656.

This research presents an integrated approach to analyzing patient characteristics, type of care (admission to a nursing home or services provided in a community setting) and patient outcomes after six months. The sample was comprised of 352 patients verified as needing intermediate care and receiving care in nursing homes, foster homes or at home through comprehensive intermediate home care services. Overall, findings suggest that patient characteristics affect patient outcomes differently in nursing home versus community intermediate care settings.

21.   Diamond, Timothy. (1992). Making Gray Gold: Narratives in Nursing Home Care. Chicago, IL: University of Chicago Press, 280 pages.

This book joins a long list of critiques of nursing home care in the United States. The author, a sociologist, has used participant observation to describe life in a nursing home through the eyes of nursing assistants and residents. The book closes with a set of recommendations designed to ameliorate the problems that the author describes.

22.   Erdman, Palmore (1987). "Total Chance of Institutionalism Among the Aged." The Gerontologist, 16(6).

This longitudinal study spanning 20 years estimates that the chance of institutionalism before death is approximately one in four. These findings differed from those of previous research in two ways; first, a lower chance of institutionalism (as compared to higher) was found among the financially disadvantaged, and second, that as an older individual ages, the prevalence rate of institutionalism rises dramatically.   The article concludes that further research and replication of these findings is necessary.

23.   George, Linda K. (1984). "The Institutionalized." In Erdman B. Palmore (Ed.) Handbook on the Aged in the United States. Westport, CT: Greenwood Press, 339-354.

The author gives a historical context to nursing homes, explains the types of institutions and the characteristics of the institutionalized aged, gives predictors and effects of institutionalization, and reviews policy issues and topics on which further research is needed.

24.   Gordon, George K. (1985). "The Social Readjustment Value of Becoming a Nursing Home Resident." The Gerontologist, 25(4):398-402.

Based on the Social Readjustment Rating Scale (SRRS) created by Momes and Rahe in 1967, the event of becoming a nursing home resident was rated in terms of perceived stress and was compared to the onset of illness. Becoming a nursing home resident was rated at 62, in comparison with the ratings of other major stressful life events: marriage (50), divorce (63) and death of a spouse (76). There are particular psychological changes in individual perception over time which limit the findings. The significance of this score needs to be further explored; it is considered surprisingly low.

25.   Greene, Vernon L. and Jan I. Ondrich. (1990). "Risk Factors for Nursing Home Admissions and Exits: A Discrete-Time Hazard Function Approach." Journal of Gerontology: Social Sciences, 45(6):S250-258.

This study used a time hazard approach to examining admissions to and exits from nursing homes. Major factors examined were ethnicity/race, age, home ownership, living alone, and presence in the community of a large proportion of nursing home beds, and richer community service environments.

26.   Gubrium, Jaber F. (1975). Living and Dying at Murray Manor. New York, NY: St. Martin's Press, 221 pages.

This book describes the social organization of a nursing home. Using the research technique of participant observation, the author, a sociologist, sought to answer the question, "How is care in a nursing home accomplished by those who participate in its everyday life?" What emerges is the picture of a complex social world that rests upon staff and resident interactions. The book should be especially valuable to the student who has spent little or no time in a nursing home and will help the experienced student to achieve greater understanding of his or her experiences.

27.   Haber, Paul A. L. (1987). "Nursing Homes" in The Encyclopedia of Aging, George L. Maddox editor-in-chief. New York, NY: Springer Publishing Co., Inc.

Nursing homes, as one of the fastest growing segments of the health care arena, have undergone and brought about major changes over the past few decades. Despite available alternatives to nursing homes, it is believed that for the next half century, nursing homes will continue to be an integral part of the long term care system. This article discusses the origin of nursing homes and the effects the passage of Medicare and Medicaid have had upon the industry. Three classes of nursing homes are described, followed by data from a survey conducted in 1979 by the Department of Health, Education, and Welfare that examined six topics;   facility, staff, financial, residence, discharge, and charge characteristics. Patient rights and the need to involve and train more health professionals in the area of geriatric care are pointed out as areas of growing interest. Finally, the coordination and involvement of a multidisciplinary health care team is recommended as the best approach to effective nursing home care.

28.   Kahana, Eva   (1987).   "Institutionalization"   in   The Encyclopedia of Aging.   George L. Maddox, editor-in-chief. New York, NY: Springer Publishing Co., Inc.

The effects and impacts of institutionalization on the 5% of the over- 65 age group who are institutionalized in this country at any one time is the focus of this article.   Highlighted are factors that heighten the probability of institutionalization, noting especially the interaction between vulnerability and dependence and the lack or inadequacy of social supports for an individual. The article points out disparities between older and more recent research regarding the effects of living in an institution. Older studies have reported the negative influences of institutional living whereas more recent literature have found positive influences to be emerging. It is suggested that changes increasing attention to residents' well-being by matching environmental characteristics with individual preferences and capabilities, will be combined with wider acceptance of institutions as part of the social community and growing sophistication of consumers, to bring about further improvement in institutions.

29.   Kane, Rosalie A. and Robert L. Kane. (1987). Long Term Care: Principles, Programs and Policies. New York, NY: Springer Publishing Co., 422 pages.

This book presents a comprehensive overview of issues in long term care. Evidence of the effects of various long term care programs compiled from decades of research and demonstration projects is reviewed. Information is provided on entitlement, financing mechanisms and quality controls. The authors provide a synthesis of reported information and recommend strategies for delivering optimal long term care.

30.   Kemper, Peter and Christopher M. Murtaugh. (1991). "Lifetime Use of Nursing Home Care." The New England Journal of Medicine, 324(9):595-600.

Data from the 1986 National Mortality Followback Survey are used to estimate the amount of time a person has spent or is projected to spend in a nursing home over a lifetime. Data analysis indicated that 37% of those who died at 65 years of age or older in 1986 had spent time in a nursing home. Projections of nursing home use by the almost 2.2 million persons who turned 65 in 1990 include that 900,000 (43%) will use a nursing home at least once before they die and that about one-third will spend at least three months (and 24% at least one year) in a nursing home. Factors which potentially could affect future nursing home use are discussed.

31.   Koff, Theodore H.   (1982).   Long Term Care: An Approach to Serving the Frail Elderly. Boston, MA: Little, Brown, and Co., 144 pages.

This book relates the history of long term care to a new concept in which services are developed and coordinated to respond to the ever-growing needs of people living with the disabling complications of chronic illness. It reviews the history of long term care, looks at current components and organization of the long term care system, discusses human resources questions, and shows how the current system can be modified to better respond to patients' needs.

32. Lawton, M. Powell, Patricia A. Parmelee and Ira R. Katz. (1991). "The Relation of Pain to Depression among Institutionalized Aged." Journal of Gerontology, 46(1):15-21.

This article explores the relationship of chronic pain and depression in the elderly who are institutionalized. Though the tendency for depressed people to report more severe pain than the non-depressed is well-documented in younger populations, this study focuses on the elderly. Data was gathered from 598 residents of a multilevel care facility. Initial analysis examined the association of pain with depression and other mood states. Further analysis explored the role of health and functional capacity that might affect the relationship between pain and depression.

33. Leibson, Cynthia et al. (1990). "Disposition at Discharge and 60-Day Mortality among Elderly People Following Shorter Hospital Stays: A Population-Based Comparison." The Gerontologist, 30(3):316-322.

This study investigates the effects of the Medicare Prospective Payment System (PPS) on mortality and hospital discharges among persons aged 65 and over who were discharged from three hospitals for each of the calendar years 1980, 1985 and 1987. Disposition at discharge was classified as either home (including self-care and home health care), nursing home, died in hospital or other. Findings indicate that sample subjects spent less time in the hospital, were at greater risk of dying within 60 days of discharge and were more often discharged to a nursing home setting in 1987 (post-PPS) than in 1980 (pre-PPS). The authors conclude that these increased risks were most likely due to post-PPS subjects being older and sicker.

34.   Moos, Rudolf H. and Christine Timko. (1991).   "A
Typology of Social Climates in Group Residential Facilities for
Older People." Journal of Gerontology, 46(3):S160-S169.

This article presents a classification of social climates arrived at
by analyzing attributes of 235 nursing homes, residential care
facilities and congregate apartments.   The study showed six
clusters based on the criteria of measurement.   Two social
climates, the supportive and the self-directed and supportive, were
well-organized and represent a humanistic environment that
emphasizes interpersonal support between residents, staff and
administration. These types of facilities scored high on cohesion,
physical comfort and independence. Facilities where there was
open conflict among these constituencies scored low on cohesion,
independence and system maintenance dimensions, as did
facilities exhibiting suppressed conflict.   The group showing
Emergent-Positive characteristics scored average and above
average on all seven dimensions. The group of facilities classified
as unresponsive scored average or below average on all seven
dimensions. The unresponsive facilities placed little emphasis on
residents' needs and preferences. Where there was an emphasis
on choice and independence, the study showed a high rating for
residents' well-being.   Conflict served to air differences but
resulted in a negative score on cohesion.

35.   Morris, Carolyn L. and Elizabeth B. Dexter. (1989).
"Taking the Clinic to the Clients: Geriatric Health in a Residential
Setting." The Gerontologist, 29(6):822-826.

This article provides a description and evaluation of the three
outreach clinics established by the Turner Geriatric Clinic under
the auspices of the Division of Geriatric Medicine of the University
of Michigan Medical School. Operating in three subsidized
high-rise residential buildings for senior citizens, the clinics use a
multidisciplinary team approach to health education, prevention,
chronic illness management and psychosocial support and
provide primary care, special services and care for minor acute
problems. Support services include meals, housekeeping, physical

therapy, occupational and activity therapy, social work services, dietary counseling, limited transportation and psychological counseling.

36.   Palmore, Erdman B. (1990). "Predictors of Outcome in Nursing Homes." The Journal of Applied Gerontology, 9(2):172-184.

The author successfully predicted length of stay and type of discharge by analyzing 22 admission characteristics In two nursing homes. The implications of these findings are discussed in this article.

37.   Qassis, Salim and Davis C. Hayden. (1990). "Effects of Environment on Psychological Well-Being of Elderly Persons." Psychological Reports, 69(1):147-149.

This study investigated the psychological well-being of older people living independently, in retirement homes and in nursing homes to examine how environment contributes to or detracts from well-being. Scales were designed for physical and social functioning. The physical scale assessed ability to bathe, dress, undress, eat, move about and brush one's teeth. The social scale assessed "the amount of visitation by relatives, friends, and neighbors, as well as time spent reading books, watching television, pursuing social interests, attending activities, exercising, and general recreation." A general well-being scale was used to assess self-representation of depression and tension anxiety.

38.   Tisdale, Sallie. (1987). Harvest Moon: Portrait of a Nursing Home. New York, NY: Henry Holt and Company, 204 pages.

This incisive case illustration offers an excellent window into the world of a nursing home as portrayed through the lives of some of its residents. The literary style used throughout conveys an easy familiarity which helps to draw the reader in, providing an intimate sense of this unique and strange environment. The author has expertly interwoven many of the difficult issues to which nursing homes and their personnel are subject in the rapidly changing field of long term care. The book should prove very informative to novice and professional alike.

39.   Vaughn, Stephanie and Shelia A. Sorrentino. (1992). OBRA Nurse Aide Skills Manual. St. Louis, MO: Mosby Year Books, 302 pages.

The authors have written a primer presenting the OBRA Nurse's Aide Training and Competency Evaluation requirements and discuss how those requirements interface with patients' needs.

40.   Wilking, Spencer and Elizabeth Markson. (1991). Social, Functional and Medical Predictors of Institutionalization: Development of a Risk Profile from the Framingham Study. Washington, DC: AARP Andrus Foundation.

This study examines the relative contributions of social, cognitive, functional and medical factors to the prospective risk of nursing home placement over a five-year period among 837 male and 1,254 female elders comprising the survivors in a general population sample of Framingham, Massachusetts. Data analysis resulted in the development of gender specific risk models. Also, the authors developed a method that enables individuals and their families to calculate the probability of their admission to a nursing home within three or five years using the Framingham data.

41.   Wingard, Deborah L., Denise Williams and Robert M. Kaplan. (1987). "Institutional Care Utilization by the Elderly: A Critical Review." The Gerontologist, 27:156-163.

The question of who utilizes nursing home care is much more complex than may appear at first glance. In this article, the authors review previous research addressing rates of utilization and factors associated with utilization of nursing home care by older persons. Emphasis is on limitations of these studies and the directions that future research should take. The article introduces the reader to the complexities of the topic, provides guidance in evaluating related studies, and illustrates some of the problems encountered in long term care research.

Mental Health Issues

42.   Bienenfeld, David and Beverly G. Wheeler. (1989). "Psychiatric Services to Nursing Homes: A Liaison Model." Hospital and Community Psychiatry, 40(8):793-794.

The authors found that more than 70% of residents of nursing homes had psychiatric disorders and that this percentage was growing. Trial programs were set up for providing treatment to these residents at outpatient clinics and within the nursing homes. An on-site program in the homes was then designed, consisting of behavioral and communicative interventions agreed upon by the nursing care coordinator, the nursing care staff and the patient, if possible.

43.   Brink, Terry L. (Ed.). (1990).   Mental Health in the Nursing Home. Binghamton, NY: Haworth Press, 226 pages.

This book focuses on the mental health of residents in nursing homes or other long term care facilities. Section one covers how to help patients and their families. Chapter topics include easing the transition to a nursing home, evaluating the functions of daily living of patients with Alzheimer's disease or other dementias, special treatment units for patients with Alzheimer's disease or other dementias, reducing excess disabilities, and generalized effects of skills training for staff upon older adults. Section two covers group therapy in the nursing home. The chapters in this section discuss the organizational logistics of running a dementia group, organizing group programs, empowering residents and building a therapeutic community through specialized groups.

44.   Cohen, Gene D. (1989). "The Interface of Mental and Physical Health Phenomena in Later Life: New Directions in Geriatric Psychiatry." Gerontology and Geriatric Education, 9(3):27-38.

This article discusses the interface of mental health and physical health. It explores how supportive counseling therapy can benefit older adults, and discusses certain physical ailments that are often connected to mental conditions.

45.   Hayes, Pamela M., Diana Lohse and Irving Bernstein. (1991). "The Development and Testing of the Hayes and Lohse Non-Verbal Depression Scale." Clinical Gerontologist, 10(3):3-11.

The Hayes and Lohse Non-Verbal Depression Scale was designed to assess older nursing home residents whose cognitive functions may be so impaired as to prevent self-reporting of depression. The authors note that depression in the elderly is often not diagnosed or treated, partly because it is often confused with dementia or cognitive impairment. This observational score should be useful to primary caregivers by helping them assess a patient's condition and sensitizing them to symptoms of depression.

46.   Leenaars, Antoon A. et al. (1991). "Knowledge about Facts and Myths of Suicide in the Elderly." Gerontology and Geriatric Education, 12(1):61-68.

Older people are the age group with the highest rate of suicide and the lowest level of awareness about suicide facts, warning signs and preventive measures.   This article discusses comprehensive measures to prevent suicide, including adjustment counseling to major life changes, bereavement counseling, peer support groups, and ways to gain access to these groups and services.

47.   Lowenthal, Richard I. and Richard A. Marranzo. (1990). "Milestoning: Evoking Memories for Resocialization through Group Reminiscence." The Gerontologist, 30(2):269-272.

A reminiscence program was developed and designed by these authors to encourage positive communication of memories among older dysfunctional nursing home residents. After comparing other studies of reminiscence therapy, particularly Butler's "life review," which deals with the presence of a major life crisis and not active psychoses, milestoning is proposed as a method of helping cognitively impaired patients. Whereas life review involves reviewing past experiences, conflict and self-confrontation, possibly resulting in sadness, in milestoning, positive memories are stimulated by a facilitator and within a group; memories are inspired, not spontaneously evoked. Pleasant memories were selected because their recall was hypothesized to increase patient interaction with others. The conclusions drawn from this study were that milestoning did encourage positive memories, which encouraged communication and, perhaps more importantly, prompted obvious changes for disturbed, withdrawn or confused patients during the sessions but did not result in long term changes.

48.   Palmore, Erdman B. (1984). "The Mentally Ill." Handbook on the Aged in the United States, edited by Erdman B. Palmore. Westport, CT: Greenwood Press.

Mental health is one of the most pressing problems of the elderly now facing our health care system. This chapter describes how stigmatization associated with mental illness historically has compounded other specific problems related to aging. Although there have been recent advances in the treatment of mental illness of the elderly, only a very small proportion of the elderly receive proper care and therapy. The article further discusses diagnostic assessment measures and treatment services and provides a list of organizations that address the issues of the mentally ill elderly and suggests areas for future research

49.   Taft, Lois B. and Milton F. Nehrke. (1990). "Reminiscence, Life Review and Ego Integrity in Nursing Home Residents." International Journal of Aging and Human Development, 30(3):189-196.

The relationship between forms of reminiscence and ego integrity was evaluated in this study, along with the use of life review. Ego's importance in the process of aging was compared with that of reminiscence because it was postulated that reminiscence may connect the past to the present and thereby improve self-image. The results revealed, unexpectedly, that the frequency of reminiscence did not significantly relate to ego integrity. However, in evaluating the use of reminiscence, it was found that using it specifically for life review seemed to improve ego integrity. Those who reported using reminiscence for life review scored higher on the measuring of ego integrity. Therefore, being involved in life-review types of reminiscence may improve an older person's quality of life, as well as ego integrity.

50.   Thornton, Susan and Janet Brotchie. (1987). "Reminiscence: A Critical Review of the Empirical Literature." British Journal of Clinical Psychology, 26:93-111.

Reminiscence about the past is seen as significant for the older person, especially in giving new meaning to an individual's life and in improving social functioning within institutions. Studies on this activity span a wide range of functions and a variety of methods. The results of the various studies are reviewed here and conclusions on reminiscence as an age-related process or an aspect of therapeutic activity are evaluated. In addition, some studies found that the dimension of memories may differ among different age groups. Others have found that older people do not reminisce more than younger people. Studies differ on the relationship between reminiscence and mood, depression or intellect. The effect of reminiscence on life satisfaction in therapy is also questioned. Generally, the conclusions from these studies show that reminiscence has a possible positive function, but its effects on therapy are questionable.

3

Community Services

Case Management Services

51.   Hennessey, Catherine H. and Michael Hennessey. (1990). "Community-Based Long Term Care for the Elderly: Evaluation Practice Reconsidered." Medical Care Review, 47(2):221-259.

Limitations of traditional, "non-system" geriatric care include fragmented coverage, inequitable access to services, a bias toward institutional care and a lack of coordination of services. These authors evaluated 13 community-based long term care (CBLTC) projects funded by HCFA that offer an alternative. All include case management and operate under Medicare and Medicaid waivers. No reduction in health care expenditures was observed. Improved life satisfaction, activity participation, quality of life, morale and social interaction were seen, and existing informal care appeared not to have been displaced.

52.   Williams, Judith K.   (1993).   "Case Management: Opportunities for Service Providers." Home Health Care Services Quarterly, 14(1):5-40.

The use of case managers in care coordination for the elderly is growing. Case management is thought to be the most effective route to delivering service with limited resources. Though there is little systematic research to support this opinion, it is widespread. Demonstration projects provide some anecdotal evidence, but few conclusions to support the rhetoric of case management. The author makes a case for flexibility of organization and sensitivity of provision.

Hospice

53.   Carey, Deborah Allen. (1984). "Home and Nature Links Highlight Hospices." Hospital, 58(4):102 and 105.

A summary of design considerations for a hospice facility is presented based on results from a study conducted by the author of 48 planned or existing architecturally distinct hospice units.

54.   Koff, Theodore H.   (1980).   Hospice: A Caring Community. Cambridge, MA: Winthrop Publishers, 196 pages.

This book is written for the student of hospice, whether a classroom student or someone working in health care. It is specifically directed to persons attempting to learn about hospice care in order to help develop or evaluate a hospice program or to adapt similar ideas to other forms of health care.

55.   Mor, Vincent, Gerry Hendershot and Cynthia Cryan. (1989). "Awareness of Hospice Services: Results of a National Survey." Public Health Reports, 104(2):178-183.

This article investigates the level of familiarity with and perceived access to hospice services among the older adult population. Data analysis was conducted on respondents to the Supplement on Aging, National Health Interview Survey, 1984, and was used to make estimates of the total U.S. non-institutionalized population aged 55 and over. Results indicate that there is a substantial reduction in level of awareness of hospice as one ages, with the oldest-old being the least familiar with the concept. Also, there appear to be regional variations in familiarity with hospice services and awareness of hospice availability. The authors suggest that future hospice use may be more strongly related to providers' rather than to the general public's knowledge and awareness of this service to the terminally ill.

Rural Issues

56. Clark, Daniel O. (1992). "Residence Differences in Formal and Informal Long Term Care." The Gerontologist, 32(2):227-233.

This study uses the cross-sectional data from the longitudinal National Long Term Care Survey (NLTCS) 1982. The initial screening consisted of 36,000 Medicare recipients who were 65 years of age or older. The study sample was comprised of 6,393 older persons who indicated having a functional disability that had lasted, or was expected to last, three months or longer. Results of this study show that when residence differences (rural versus urban) in informal assistance with ADLs and IADLs were compared, a lower percentage of non-institutionalized disabled residents of rural areas received formal assistance than did their urban counterparts. Because rural older adults receive less formal assistance does not mean they are disadvantaged or have a high unmet need for care compared to urban dwellers. Results indicate no statistically significant differences across rural and urban areas regarding unmet need for assistance even after controlling for the level of impairment and socio-demographic characteristics.

57. Krout, John. (1991). Case Management for the Rural Elderly: A National Analysis. Washington, DC: AARP Andrus Foundation, 156 pages.

This study provides a descriptive overview of case management in rural areas across the nation. Data was collected and analyzed on 555 agencies (representing 51% of the agencies identified by telephone calls to each state). Information on the following case management characteristics were collected: core agency activities, staff, resources, mandates, licensure, target populations and quality assurance, as well as other operational and policy issues.

58.   Nyman, John A., Anindya Sen, Benjamin Y. Chan and Paul P. Commins. (1991). "Urban/Rural Differences In Home Health Patients and Services." The Gerontologist, 31(4):457-466.

Data from the 1988-89 Wisconsin Annual Survey of Home Health Agencies were used to determine whether an urban location implies a greater tendency to use home health care. In this study, evidence suggests that urban residents are more likely than their rural counterparts to be home health clients. Results indicate that urban dwellers are more likely to correspond to the typical long term care patient, especially in their dependencies and the length of time that they receive services. Conversely, rural patients more closely fit a post-acute pattern, recovering from chronic diseases. The authors caution that to ascertain whether access to services is a major problem in rural areas research must go beyond comparing services in urban versus rural settings and explore differences and similarities between patient needs and life-style.

59.   Pearson-Scott, Jean and Karen A. Roberto. (1987). "Informal Supports of Older Adults: A Rural-Urban Comparison." Family Relations, 36:444-449.

This comparative research study was conducted to examine similarities and differences between urban and rural older adults on exchanges of assistance and social activities with children and friends. From 1980 to 1981, two data sets were initiated in the same Southwest location: 1) an urban sample of 180 white adults aged 65 to 90 years, and 2) a rural sample of 145 white adults 65 to 89 years of age. In-person interviews were conducted with sample respondents. Background variables (marital status, income, age, health, etc.) and the morale of respondents were assessed. Also, the extent of helping behaviors and social activity/interaction between respondents, friends and families were measured. Significantly, a greater proportion of rural females than of urban females received assistance from children when they were ill. With the exception of urban older adults, social activities with friends and support network variables had no significant influence on the morale of older persons in the sample. Friendships among rural area adults tended to involve more instrumental qualities and fewer leisure/social qualities than occur among urban dwelling adults. Findings indicate the significance of involving rural and urban older adult support networks in care decisions related to the health and well-being of older adults.

60.   Revicki, Dennis A. and Jim P. Mitchell. (1990). "Strain, Social Support and Mental Health In Rural Elderly Individuals." Journal of Gerontology: Social Sciences, 45(6):S267-274.

This study investigated the role of different dimensions of social support in the life strain-psychological distress relationship of 240 rural adults aged 65 years or older, randomly selected from the patient population of a family practice clinic. Measures of socio-emotional support, instrumental support and social contacts were used to examine the relationships among social support and multiple indicators of chronic life strain and mental health. ADL impairment and illness disability were found to be strongly associated with emotional distress and life satisfaction. Physical health status was found to be the source of life strain that most affected perceptions of life satisfaction and psychological distress. Also, effective instrumental support and social contacts moderated the relationship between life strain and mental health in older persons.

61.   Shaughnessy, Peter W., Robert E. Schlenker and Herbert A. Silverman. (1988). "Evaluation of the National Swing-Bed

Program in Rural Hospitals." Health Care Financing Review, 10(1):87-94.

This is a general overview of the swing-bed program, which is designed to allow rural hospitals to provide services to relatively short stay long term care patients. These patients are difficult to place in community nursing homes due to their intense need for medical treatment. Swing-bed patients have shorter stays and greater rehabilitation potential than their nursing home counterparts. Their conditions tend to be sub-acute conditions such as recovery from surgery, hip fractures and need for catheters. This program allows hospitals with low acute care occupancy rates and a large elderly population to utilize their excess capacity to offer labor-intensive services to residents of their local area.

62.   Williams, Frank G., Ellen Netting and Pamela Hood-Szivek. (1988). "Developing Swing-Bed Programs In Rural Arizona Hospitals." The Gerontologist, 28(4):495-498.

This article discusses the development of six swing-bed programs In rural Arizona hospitals. Goals included assistance to develop a continuum of care, to assist patients to remain within the community throughout their medical treatment, to facilitate recovery and rehabilitation through the encouragement of informal networks of family and neighbors, and to assist rural hospitals to recruit trained geriatric care staff. After implementation, several hospitals said that this program would probably make the difference between survival and closure for their institutions.

Service Utilization

63.   Ezell, Mark and John W. Gibson. (1989). "The Impact of Informal Social Networks on the Elderly's Need for Services." Journal of Gerontological Social Work, 14(3/4):3-18.

This study examined the relationship between current and anticipated service needs and available informal support assistance for 75 community dwelling adults age 60 years and older. Findings demonstrate that almost all of the sample (96%) reported that help would be available from a friend or relative if they became sick or disabled. Respondents anticipated needing many more services in the future than they were currently receiving. Periodic health screening, emergency response, chores and friendly visiting were more often selected than any other of the 18 services included in the survey. Although the data were not statistically significant, subjects without informal support networks expressed both a greater current and anticipated future need for services than persons who had informal assistance.

64.   Koff, Theodore H. (1988). New Approaches to Health Care for an Aging Population: Developing a Continuum of Chronic Care Services. San Francisco, CA: Jossey-Bass Publishers, 270 pages.

The multiple chronic conditions that proliferate as one ages are not adequately acknowledged or dealt with by the current acute-care-centered systems. By the year 2000, those over age 65 in this country will account for 50% of all health care expenditures. This book uses in-depth studies of five successful chronic care systems for the elderly to detail the necessary steps involved in planning, implementing and administering a coordinated program of chronic care services. These systems show why the use of a continuum of services is the most effective response to chronic illness.

65.   Wolinsky, Fredric and Robert J. Johnson. (1991). "The Use of Health Services by Older Adults." Journal of Gerontology: Social Sciences, 46(6):S345-357.

This research study used baseline data from the Longitudinal Study on Aging to estimate, cross-sectionally, the relationships in the behavioral model of health services utilization which views the use of health services as a function of the predisposing, enabling and need characteristics of the individual. Results indicate that need characteristics are the principal determinants of health service utilization. The author cautions that the findings do not characterize the health care system as equitable. Important health care utilization characteristics which have been absent from previous research studies are identified.

Chronic Illness

66.   Chronic Disease and Disability: Beyond the Acute Medical Model. (1990). Sponsored by The Pew Charitable Trust, 105 pages.

The five papers that comprise this volume were produced to serve as a catalyst for broader discussion at a Pew Health Policy Program annual meeting. Each author focuses on an issue relevant to enhancing our nation's ability to meet the challenge of chronic illness, including system building, the transition of acute care into chronic care models, post-acute and long term care financing and delivery, employer initiatives in long term care and issues of prevention.

67.   Kerson, Toba S. with Lawrence A. Kerson. (1985). Understanding Chronic Illness: The Medical and Psychosocial Dimensions of Nine Diseases. New York, NY: The Free Press, 369 pages.

The authors discuss nine debilitating, chronic illnesses: arthritis, cancer, dementia, diabetes, epilepsy, heart disease, respiratory illness, stroke and substance abuse. The medical characteristics, typical stages and symptoms, diagnostic and treatment procedures, outcomes of treatment and psychosocial impacts are discussed for these diseases. In addition, legal and practical issues affecting the life of the chronically ill person are presented. Directories of self-help groups and relevant government agencies are included.

68.   Lubkin, Ilene Morof. (1986). <u>Chronic Illness: Impact and Interventions</u>. Boston, MA: Jones and Bartlett Publishers, Inc., 395 pages.

This book looks at the issues of chronic illness from the perspective of its effects upon the lives of the individual and the family. The goal of the author is to help health professionals educate the chronically ill and members of their support networks in long term self-management, thereby enhancing their quality of life.

69.   Strauss, Anselm and Juliet M. Corbin. (1988). <u>Shaping a New Health Care System: The Explosion of Chronic Illness as a Catalyst for Change</u>. San Francisco, CA: Jossey-Bass Publishers, 176 pages.

This book addresses the need for changes in the present health care system in response to the increasing numbers of chronically ill people in our society. The prevalence and nature of chronic illness is reviewed, as is the history of how chronic illness has been handled. Approaches, models and implications for future health care are outlined at the end of the book.

4

Administrative Issues

Patient Care

70.   Biegel, David E., Marcia K. Petchers, Arlene Snyder and Beverly Beisgen. (1989). "Unmet Needs and Barriers to Service Delivery for the Blind and Visually Impaired Elderly." <u>The Gerontologist</u>, <u>29</u>:86-91.

This study examined the extent to which lack of integration between aging network agencies and blindness agencies may result in an under-served blind and visually impaired older population. A survey of local aging and blindness services in Pennsylvania indicated a lack of communication between the two networks. Unmet needs identified by aging and blindness services staff included accessibility, specialized services, social/recreational and educational opportunities. The authors make recommendations for addressing these problems.

71.   Kemp, Margaret G. (1990). <u>Preventing Pressure Sores in the Elderly</u>. Washington, DC: AARP Andrus Foundation, 5 pages.

The purpose of this research was to identify indicators to predict the clinical effectiveness of pressure-reducing devices for decreasing the risk of developing pressure sores. The sample consisted of 84 persons aged 65 years and older who were newly-admitted patients on general medical units in a tertiary care medical center, an acute geriatric medical unit and a long term care facility. Patients who did not have a pressure sore but were determined to be at risk for developing one (as assessed using the Braden Scale for Predicting Pressure Sore Risk) were admitted to the study. Results indicate that interface pressure was not useful in predicting the clinical effectiveness of the two pressure reducing devices studied. However, Braden Scores were statistically relevant as predictors of risk and were recommended to be part of a standard protocol for preventing pressure sores.

72.   Koff, Theodore H. (1986). "Wellness and Long Term Care." In Wellness and Health Promotion for the Elderly, Ken Dychtwald, editor. Rockville, MD: Aspen Systems Corporation, 119-132.

The author suggests that the concept of wellness has not been well-integrated into the coordinated continuum of services that currently defines the long term care system. Some of the issues outlined in this chapter describe ways by which wellness can be incorporated into the continuum and include the cultivation of a better understanding of the preventive benefits of lifetime health practices and the utility of the hospice model to enable caregivers to begin to deal with the person as a whole. The book argues for the importance of turning around the popular conception of long term care as dealing only with illness, disability, or limitations by learning to conceptualize and teach about long term care in terms of wellness and adaptability.

73.   Palmer, Robert M. (1990). "Failure to Thrive in the Elderly: Diagnosis and Management." Geriatrics, 45(9):47-55.

Failure to thrive (FTT) is defined as "a gradual decline in physical or cognitive function of an older person, usually accompanied by weight loss and social withdrawal that occurs without immediate explanation." FTT is a common occurrence in institutionalized and hospitalized older adults. The earlier FTT is diagnosed, the lower are the chances of further decline, unnecessary hospitalization or death. Although older persons are predisposed to FTT for reasons such as impaired senses, social isolation, inadequate social supports and age-associated diseases, symptoms associated with FTT may be seen as normal attributes of aging, not an identifiable, treatable, illness.

74.   Vourlekis, Betsy S., Donald E. Gelfand and Roberta R. Greene. (1992). "Psychosocial Needs and Care in Nursing Homes: Comparison of Views of Social Workers and Home Administrators." The Gerontologist, 32(1):113-119.

OBRA regulations implemented on October 1, 1990 require all facilities to assess medically-related social and emotional needs of each resident and provide a social worker in each facility of 120 beds or more. This article examines these needs and care provided from the view of the social worker and administrators.

Gerontological Nursing

75.   Gallo, Joseph J., William Reichel and Lillian Anderson. (1988). Handbook of Geriatric Assessment. Rockville, MD: Aspen Publishers, Inc., 231 pages.

This book is a guide for practitioners in multidimensional geriatric assessment. The authors promote the use of comprehensive evaluations of mental, physical, psychological, functional, social and economic factors. Information is provided on assessing the value of the history of the older patient. Criteria for the organization and assessment of geriatric programs is provided.

76.   Matteson, Mary Ann and Eleanor S. McConnell. (1988). Gerontological Nursing: Concepts and Practice. Philadelphia, PA: W. B. Saunders Co., 857 pages.

This comprehensive textbook covers the full range of topics necessary for a complete understanding of gerontological nursing. The authors begin with an overview of gerontological nursing, proceed to discussions of the physiological changes in the body's various functional systems that occur due to aging, and give overviews of psychosocial aging changes, clinical science considerations and the issues surrounding care settings. This book is an excellent training resource for administrators and for those they supervise.

77.   Osgood, Nancy, J. (1992). "Environmental Factors in Suicide in Long Term Care Facilities." Suicide and Life-Threatening Behavior, 22(1):98-106.

This study was conducted to identify environmental factors that were related to suicide among residents of long term care facilities.   The author distinguishes between overt suicide and indirect life-threatening behavior (ILTB).   Overt suicide includes wrist-slashing, jumping, hanging, shooting and asphyxiation. ILTB is defined as acts that result in physical harm that could bring about premature death, such as refusing to eat or drink, refusing to follow medical regimens or to take medications.   The study looks at four environmental factors that affect quality of care and patient outcomes in an institutional setting.

78.   Williams, T. Franklin. (1990). "Geriatrics: A Perspective on Quality of Life and Care for Older People." In Bert Spilker (Ed.) Quality of Life Assessments in Clinical Trials. New York, NY: Raven Press, Ltd.

This chapter reviews the important factors associated with quality of life and care, how they interrelate and approaches for their adequate recognition and assessment.   The quality of life characteristics determined or influenced by older adults themselves (life-style factors, screening and early detection of potential problems) as well as the psychological, social and economic factors affecting quality of life are discussed. The author defines what high quality of care for older persons is and examines specific features of its application to older persons needing care. Strategies for assessing and accomplishing high quality care are presented.

Staffing

79.   Allen, James E. (1990). "National Standards for the Licensure of Nursing Home Administrators: What Should Be Sought?" The Gerontologist, 30(5):650-657.

Data from the National Association of Boards of Examiners for Nursing Home Administrator (NAB) for all years from 1970 to 1987 were analyzed and comparisons of those from 1976 and 1987 are presented. The number of licensed nursing home administrators increased from 29,425 in 1976 to 36,724 in 1986, an increase of 25% over the decade. The largest percentage rises occurred in Alaska, Arizona, Nevada, Florida, Arkansas and Alabama. Current trends in national standards for licensure are discussed, including educational requirements and administrator in training program for original licensure, state and national examinations, continuing education for relicensure requirements and reciprocity. Possible future directions for the field are addressed, such as imposing uniform national standards, continuing the status quo, and eliminating the federal requirement for licensed nursing home administrators. The author recommends possible solutions to such unsolved problems facing the field as barriers to professional adequacy, reciprocity and access to the profession.

80.   Breser, Kathleen Pearl, Barbara A. Almanza and Robert E. Hurley. (1992). "Dietitians in Continuing Care Retirement

Communities: Workload and Overload." Journal of the American
Dietetic Association, 92(4):481-482.

Increased affluence among older persons and the increased
awareness of preventive health care result in good nutrition
becoming the norm for retirement communities. OBRA '87
included new guidelines for a minimum level of dietetic services
to retirement communities. Interviews with 26 executive directors
of continuing care retirement communities revealed there were
standards for minimal hours of providing dietary services where
high numbers of residents were served every day. The level of
services provided were evaluated with regard to size, age or type
of facility (profit/nonprofit) as well as accreditation and food
service, all of which were discussed in further detail. Food
service was also evaluated as to its role in helping to create a
better sense of community at the facility. This study suggests that
the overall success of the organization can be related to better
nutrition programs and regular services.

81.   Caudill, Marian E. and Maxine Patrick.   (1991-92).
"Turnover among Nursing Assistants: Why They Leave and Why
They Stay." The Journal of Long Term Care Administration,
19(4):29-31, Winter.

In recent literature, turnover rates as high as 75% have been
reported for nursing assistants in long term care facilities. This
survey was conducted to identify the characteristics that would
influence nursing assistants' length of stay. In general, the data
from the 996 completed surveys showed that nursing assistants
who were planning to leave were younger, had spent less time in
their current position, were paid less and were better educated
than average. Comments volunteered by participants revealed
they were interested in providing good care to their patients and
would like training to increase their skills.

82.   Deitzer, Diane, Jill Wessell, Katheryn Myles and Pamela
Trimble. (1992). "Agency Nurses: The Right Solution to Staffing

Problems?" <u>The Journal of Long Term Care Administration</u>, <u>20</u>(3):29-38, Fall.

The nursing shortage has hit long term care facilities particularly hard. The solution to this problem is often agency nurses. The study reported in this article compares two similar facilities to examine the use of non-facility nurses in light of OBRA '87 dictates. The study was conducted through interviews. It was concluded that although the nursing shortage will require continued use of nursing pools, this is an expensive approach.

83.   Fanale, James E. (1989). "The Nursing Home Medical Director." <u>Journal of the American Geriatrics Society</u>, <u>37</u>(4):369-375.

The role of the medical director in nursing homes has never been adequately defined or standardized. This article offers an insight into this issue and addresses some of the problems that militate against effective leadership in this vital position. Successful assumption of the director's role is shown to lie not only in active participation on the administrative team, but also in the ability to act as a strong liaison with the local medical community and other long term care professionals in the community.

84.   Kelly, Marsha K. (1989). "The Omnibus Budget Reconciliation Act of 1987: A Policy Analysis." <u>Nursing Clinics of North America</u>, <u>24</u>(3):791-794.

This author looks at how OBRA '87 impacts the staffs of nursing homes and how it will force staff members to take primary responsibility for quality of service delivery.

85.   Pillemer, Karl and David W. Moore. (1989). "Abuse of Patients in Nursing Homes: Findings from a Survey of Staff." <u>The Gerontologist</u>, <u>29</u>(3):314-319.

This survey was designed to assess the scope and nature of physical and psychological abuse in nursing homes through querying a random sample of registered nurses, licensed practical nurses, and nurse's aides. Respondents were asked to report abusive actions they had witnessed or had committed. The results showed that 36% of the sample had seen at least one incident of physical abuse and 81% had witnessed psychological abuse during the preceding year. The strongest predictors of abuse were situational variables concerning the staff.

86.   Shore, Herbert, Marvin Ernst and Shawn Nix. (1988). Sensitizing People to the Processes of Aging: the In-Service Educator's Guide, Second Edition.   Denton, TX: Center for Studies in Aging, University of North Texas, 132 pages.

Originally intended as an in-service educator's guide, this book, which deals with the importance of understanding the relationship between the sensory processes and aging, quickly gained a much wider audience as an educational tool for working with older persons. The revised edition provides guidance in organizing and conducting training programs for persons who are working or will work with older persons but who have little or no formal training in gerontology. Included are suggestions for simulating sensory loss as a training technique, other training resources and an extensive bibliography.

87.   Tellis-Nayak, V. and Mary Tellis-Nayak. (1989). "Quality of Care and the Burden of Two Cultures: When the World of the Nurse's Aide Enters the World of the Nursing Home."   The Gerontologist, 29(3):307-313.

The findings in this study suggest that turnover in nurse's aides in nursing homes is a result of cultural influences that cannot be separated from their work experience. Nurse's aides mostly come from lower-income families, have little education, are mostly women, are low skilled and poorly paid. Nursing homes are cold, impersonal and heartless institutions that have little time to deal with a nurse's aide's personal problems. The aides learn to keep their distance from both professional staff and from patients. This leads to their making residents targets of their discontent. Without an institutional structure that understands this, patients suffer because of the frustrations of their caregivers.

88.   Waxman, Howard M., Erwin A. Carner and Gale Berkenstock. (1984). "Job Turnover and Job Satisfaction among Nursing Home Aides." The Gerontologist, 24(5):503-509.

Annual turnover among nursing home aides is between 40% and 75%. This study looked at the possibility that turnover may be related to nursing home management style. The results showed that highly structured management systems had higher turnover than homes that allowed employee input to decision-making.

Quality Assurance

89.   Lemke, Sonne and Rudolf H. Moos. (1989). "Ownership and Quality of Care in Residential Facilities for the Elderly." The Gerontologist, 29(2):209-215.

The purpose of this study was to determine whether ownership of a facility (proprietary, nonprofit or Veterans Administration) made a difference in the quality of care received. The authors concluded: 1) the quality of care in privately-owned nursing home facilities suffers because owners try so hard to make a profit for shareholders; 2) nonprofit nursing facilities are able to stretch patient dollars farther because they do not have shareholders to pay; and 3) government-owned nursing homes provide poor quality care because they are not subject to competition like privately-owned and nonprofit facilities.

90.   Glass, Anne P. (1992). "Nursing Home Quality: The Administrator's Responsibility." The Journal of Long Term Care Administration, 31-36, Winter.

The author reviews the literature and provides a framework identifying factors influencing nursing home quality. The greatest impact is generated by the commitment, attitudes and policy of the administrator and supervisory nursing staff. A quality framework for administrators is provided as well as guidance about which of the quality factors are controllable.

91.   Gustafson, David H., Francois C. Sainfort, Richard Van Konigsveld and David R. Zimmerman. (1990). "The Quality Assessment Index for Measuring Nursing Home Quality." Health Services Research, 25(1):97-125.

There has been a lot of concern over defining, measuring and assuring quality of care in nursing homes. This article presents characteristics that should be included in measuring quality of care. It also describes an index designed to measure quality of care. Several tests were done to measure the validity and reliability of the index; those results are also reported in this article.

92.   Nyman, John A. (1989). "Excess Demand, Consumer Rationality and the Quality of Care in Regulated Nursing Homes." Health Services Research, 24(1):105-124.

This study investigated whether nursing homes take advantage of irrational or confused patients by providing an inadequate quality of care. Measurement of care quality is based on Medicaid code violations, since noncompliance with codes would be a serious concern for patients, if they knew about it, and an indicator that other undesirable characteristics may be present. Data used in this study came from Wisconsin's 1983 Annual Survey of Nursing Homes. The sample consisted of 260 nursing homes. The average number of beds per home was 133.4 with an average number of empty beds of 6.8.

93.   Shaughnessy, Peter W., Robert E. Schlenker and Andrew M. Kramer. (1990). "Quality of Long Term Care in Nursing Homes and Swing-Bed Hospitals." Health Services Research, 25(1):65-94.

This article compares the quality of long term care in swing-bed hospitals with the quality of nursing home care. Patient outcomes as well as structural and process measures of quality were used to measure quality. Swing-bed hospitals and nursing homes do not serve the same types of patients and therefore complement each other rather than compete. The study questions whether one is better than the other.

94.   Tellis-Nayak, V., JoAnn Day and David J. Ward. (1988). Nursing Home Exemplars of Quality. Springfield, IL: Charles C. Thomas, 207 pages.

Unlike nursing home literature replete with descriptions of poor and abusive care of residents, the research reported in this book concentrated on eight Illinois homes identified as providing a high-quality care. Quality care is defined in Part I, the eight homes are described in Part II. Each of the six chapters of Part III describes a key factor in achieving high quality care.

Functional Status

95.   Calhoun, Donald W. and Lipman, Aaron (1984). "The Disabled" in Handbook on the Aged in the United States," Erdman B. Palmore, editor. Westport, CT: Greenwood Press.

This chapter provides a thought-provoking definition of disability as it relates to aging. By its nature, aging is accompanied by an increasing disabling conditions that tend to increase in severity. This chapter discusses physical impairment, and issues of stigmatization, isolation, and dependency. It also describes the effects of disability on sexuality. Barriers to health maintenance and nutrition are pointed out. The final chapter reviews issues of long term care provided to the disabled elderly by institutions or other community alternatives.

96.   Kane, Robert L. and Rosalie A. Kane (1982). <u>Values and Long Term Care</u>. Lexington, MA: D. C. Heath and Company.

Chapters in this book explore the emergence of assessment of health status and of value preferences in long term care policy and practice. Topics include measurement approaches, practical approaches, and ways to measure value preferences.

97.   Koff, Theodore H. "Long Term Care Assessment" (1987) in <u>The Encyclopedia of Aging,</u> George L. Maddox, editor-in-chief. New York , NY: Springer Publishing Co., Inc.,

In addition to discussing benefits and concerns regarding comprehensive multidisciplinary assessment of long term care raised by other researchers, this article points out both a need for assessment in the area of social policy, where it could influence planning, availability, and access to services and the area of assessment of the individual and the family or support network to identify strengths that may contribute to functional improvement, increase caregiver sensitivity, and identify tools and resources to aid and encourage the maintenance of wellness. Additionally, assessment can help the individual understand the influence of the environment upon wellness, and can provide protection from misdiagnosis and inappropriate care. Furthermore, only after a comprehensive assessment is complete can an appropriate match of needs and services be achieved.

98.   Speare, Alden, Roger Avery and Leora Lawton. (1991). "Disability, Residential Mobility and Changes in Living Arrangements." <u>Journal of Gerontology: Social Sciences</u>, <u>46</u>(3):S133-142.

This article examines the relationship between health and disability and its impact on three types of living arrangements of older persons: moving to a new location, living with adults other than spouse or entering an institution. Data for the study were obtained from telephone interviews conducted with 5,151 subjects (or a proxy) from the 1984-86 Longitudinal Study of Aging, National Institute on Aging. Findings reveal that need for institutionalization is strongly related to the level of care required, as indicated by degree of disability, confusion and poor health status. Duration of residence was a strong predictor of willingness to move; homeowners and persons living at the same residence 15 or more years were least likely to move.

99.   Spector, William D.   (1990).   "Functional Disability Scales."   In Bert Spilker (Ed.) Quality of Life Assessments in Clinical Trials. New York, NY: Raven Press, Ltd., 115-129.

The author reviews several functional disability scales, emphasizing scales that measure either activities of daily living or instrumental activities of daily living. The examination of each scale is divided into six sections: description, purpose and use, scale structure, reliability, validity and responsiveness. The scales have received acceptance in the clinical and research arenas and vary in terms of the quality and extent of their reliability and validity.   Important differences are highlighted and conceptual concerns are discussed.

100.   Worobey, Jacqueline L. and Ronald J. Angel. (1990). "Functional Capacity and Living Arrangements of Unmarried Elderly Persons."   Journal of Gerontology: Social Sciences, 45(3):S95-101.

This article explores the functional capacity and living arrangements of 2,498 persons aged 70 years or older who participated in the national Longitudinal Study on Aging in 1984 and were still alive in 1986. At time of follow-up, the proportion of respondents reporting problems with at least one ADL increased from 30.5% in 1984 to 42.6% in 1986. The majority of subjects whose functional capacity declined during the time period 1984-86 continued to live alone. The authors emphasize the strong preference of older persons to live alone, a propensity they predict will grow even stronger among members of the baby-boom generation who have grown up in smaller families and had more privacy. Also, the implications of increased desire for independent living arrangements on the part of future generations of older women and ethnic minorities are discussed.

Environmental Design

101.   Bush-Brown, Albert and Dianne Davis (Eds.). (1992). Hospitable Design for Health Care and Senior Communities. New York, NY: Van Nostrand Reinhold, 263 pages.

This volume is made up of 93 essays by 60 authors. Some are as brief as a paragraph and others are several pages long. Linking these diverse contributions is a strong commitment to the belief that "hospitable design" is important to the well-being of older persons in a wide range of settings, from community centers and hotel conversions to adult day care and Alzheimer's units. The essays describe examples of good design in these settings and are enhanced by the liberal inclusion of drawings and photographs. The book offers nursing home administrators many challenging ideas about design.

102.   Clark, Richard C. (1984). "Market Needs Mold Nursing Home Mission for an Older Hospital." Hospitals, 58(4):96 and 98.

This article reports on a phased renovation program for a New York City hospital to accommodate skilled, intermediate and specialty care services. An "X" pattern nursing home design was used. Before and after photographs of a nursing station, patient rooms and a solarium are presented.

103.   Collins, Daniel F.   (1984).   "Skilled Nursing Unit Fashioned from Acute Care Space." Hospitals, 58(4):100.

A summary of the design goals of a acute care facility's conversion of three inpatient wings and a delivery suite into a 39-bed skilled nursing unit is presented.

104.   Nabelek, Anna K., Frances M. Tucker and Tomasz R. Letowski. (1991). "Toleration of Background Noises." Journal of Speech and Hearing Research, 34:679-685.

This study examined the effects of background noises on five groups of persons with different levels of hearing loss and hearing-aid use. Each group was tested for tolerance to six different levels of background noises ranging from babbling and traffic noise to music and a drill. Data analysis revealed that in three areas -- music, traffic noise and noise of average speech -- full-time hearing-aid users tolerated higher levels of noise than did part-time hearing-aid users or the hearing-impaired who did not use a hearing aid.

105.   Raschko, Bettyann B. (1982). Housing Interiors for the Disabled and Elderly. New York, NY: Van Nostrand Reinhold, 360 pages.

The author reviewed research that has been done on ways to make activities of daily living easier through considered design, a subject somewhat neglected in recent findings. Because In-depth understanding of varying degrees of disability is required to create housing that enhances rather than hinders the lives of those who are disabled and older, this book looks at each living space in detail and suggests ways to accomplish that goal.

106.   Roenfeld, Norman with Ann Wyatt. (1984). "Urban Nursing Home Rescued and Renovated."   Hospitals, 58(4):109-110.

A summary is given of design elements used in renovating a 75-year-old nursing home in Greenwich Village, NY.

107.   Rosenfeld, Zachary.   (1993).   "A New Approach to Nursing Home Layout and Work Patterns." Pride Institute Journal, 24-30, Winter.

New approaches to nursing home design attempt to influence treatment outcomes through resident-centered care. New facilities should include ample room for wheelchairs, therapy that can be brought to the residents, nurse's aides located close to the bedchambers and integration of total quality management into the structural design. Specific designs are discussed.

108.   Stevens and Wilkinson Architects, Engineers, Planners, Inc. (1982). "Nursing Home Design Focuses on Personal Needs of Residents." Hospitals, 56(4):126-127.

This article describes the "Y" shaped design for a three-story 150 bed nursing home as an addition to an acute care facility. Each branch of the "Y" houses 25 residents.   Patient room configurations are modular in design, with each semiprivate room flanked by two private units, shortening the distance to the nursing station. The branches of the "Y"-shaped facility converge at an area on each resident floor which includes the nursing station, a dining area and a lounge. Photographs and area drawings are presented.

109.   Thomas, Julia and Michael L. Bobrow.   (1984). "Targeting the Elderly in Facility Design." Hospitals, 58(4):83-88.

This article explores alternative care options for hospitals, both on the hospital campus and in the community. Brief descriptions of each of the following care environments are provided: Connecticut Hospice, Branford, CT; West Valley Towers (low-cost elderly housing), Van Nuys, CA; Medical Center of Delray, Delray

Beach, FL (campus care); the Motion Picture and Television Fund Country House, Woodland Hills, CA (life care); and the Kendal Retirement Community (life care). Design considerations for older persons are discussed.

Patients' Rights

110.   Annas, George J. (1989). The Rights of Patients: The Basic ACLU Guide to Patient Rights, Second Edition. Carbondale, IL: Southern Illinois University Press, 312 pages.

This second edition of an excellent overview of a person's rights in the health care system was published in cooperation with the American Civil Liberties Union. Some of the crucial areas covered include informed consent, privacy and confidentiality, the role of the patient rights advocate, a model patient bill of rights, living wills and durable powers of attorney. Primarily a reference for patients, their families and health care providers, it has also been an excellent textbook for students.

111.   Cohen-Mansfield, Jiska, Janet A. Droge and Nathan Billig. (1991). "The Utilization of the Durable Power of Attorney for Health Care among Hospitalized Elderly Patients." Journal of the American Geriatrics Society, 39(12):1174-1178.

In-person interviews with 97 hospital patients aged 64 years and older to explore the potential use of the durable power of attorney for health care (DPAHC) revealed that, of the patients interviewed, about 16% had already executed a DPAHC, another approximately 46% wanted to execute one, 47% did not want to and 8% were undecided. Over half of the respondents had not discussed their feelings about health care decisions with anyone. Respondents who had or wanted to execute a DPAHC scored higher on a cognitive test. Quality of life scores were much higher for those who had executed a DPAHC than for any other group. A three-month follow-up of the 70 patients who had not had a DPAHC indicated that only six (12%) had executed one in the interim since hospitalization. Four possible reasons for limited use of DPAHC by older adults are discussed..

112.   Doukas, David J. and Howard Brody. (1992). "After the Cruzan Case: The Primary Care Physician and the Use of Advance Directives." Journal of the American Board of Family Practice, 5(2):201-205.

This discussion of the legal ramifications of proxy decisions and advance directives for primary care physicians gives a case synopsis and explores the implications of the Cruzan case. It outlines ways in which health care practitioners can begin to discuss the use of advance directives with patients and briefly explains different methods of advance directives.

113.   Greco, Peter J., Kevin A. Schulman, Risa Lavizzo-Mourey and John Hansen-Flaschen. (1991)."The Patient Self-Determination Act and the Future of Advance Directives." Annals of Internal Medicine, 115(8):639-643.

This article outlines the contents of the 1990 Patient Self-Determination Act requiring health care settings to develop written policies concerning advance directives. It includes the steps necessary to implement the law, identifies certain limitations, and offers several approaches in promoting the preparation of advance directives. It also suggests an approach to treatment decisions when the patient's wishes are not known.

114.   High, Dallas M. (1991). "A New Myth about Families of Older People." The Gerontologist, 31(5):611-618.

A myth is emerging in the 1990s to the effect that families are inappropriate and unfit to serve as surrogate decision-makers. This article argues that the emphasis on advance directives ignores intergenerational interdependence and imposes legalistic solutions on moral issues. Public policy recommendations are also discussed.

115.   Rouse, Fenella. (1991). "The Role of State Legislatures After Cruzan: What Can--and Should--State Legislatures Do?" Law, Medicine and Health Care, 19(1/2):83-90.

Five approaches to medical decision-making are identified, with expanded treatment of situations where neither written instructions nor a designated responsible person is available or when personal wishes cannot be known. The article analyzes how courts have addressed these situations in light of the Cruzan case. The complexity and diversity of state laws can lead to impractical resolutions of crises. The author advocates a uniform comprehensive law permitting advance directives, appointment of health care proxies, authorization for someone who knew an incompetent person well to make decisions. She also suggests legislative actions that could accomplish this goal.

116.   Schwarz, Judith Kennedy. (1992). "Living Wills and Health Care Proxies: Nurse Practice Implications." Nursing and Health Care, 13(2):92-96.

This article discusses living wills and durable powers of attorney, identifying the limitations of each relative to the health care delivery system. The trend toward states' enacting laws that permit appointed agents to make medical decisions for those deemed incapacitated by a physician is examined. The New York State Health Care Act, which permits a competent adult to appoint an agent to make health care decisions, is an example; The article focuses on implications of such a law for nursing and for patient control of treatment decision-making.

117.   Wanzer, Sidney H. et al. (1989). "The Physician's Responsibility toward Hopelessly Ill Patients: A Second Look." The New England Journal of Medicine, 320(13):611-618.

The emphasis of this article is on the value of a sensitive approach to patient care. This means being knowledgeable about the different settings for dying. The article also addresses critical issues like pain and suffering, assisted suicide, euthanasia, and the importance of flexible care in a way that may be helpful for health professionals at any level.

Management

118.   Bentley, David W. and Lois Cheney. (1990). "Infection Control in the Nursing Home: The Physician's Role." Geriatrics, 45(11):59-66.

A nursing home's system for infection control structure should include a manager in charge of infection control and a committee of employees.   Employee health programs should inform employees about their role in prevention of infection. A communication mechanism should be in place to let local hospitals provide infection histories for patients transferred from one facility to another.

119.   Goldsmith, Seth B. (Ed.). (1993). Long Term Care Administration Handbook. Gaithersburg, MD: Aspen Publishers, Inc., 562 pages.

This long term care resource manual is compiled from contributions of administrators of long term care programs. A wide range of information is presented: the history of long term care, psychological and mental health issues, the role of the medical director, delivery of nursing care, ethical and caregiver issues, development and marketing functions, aspects of management and governing boards, employment issues, computer applications, quality issues, financing and fund-raising, dementia units, social work departments, activities programs, adult day care services, food services, pastoral roles, durable medical equipment, assisted living environments and architectural design.

Planning, development and implementation of programs and services are discussed.

120.   Gordon, George K. and Ruth Stryker (Eds.).   (1988). Creative Long Term Care Administration, Second Edition. Springfield, IL: Charles C. Thomas, 335 pages.

This book is composed of 24 chapters to which 13 authors have contributed. Although several of the chapters deal with topics that might be covered in a conventional textbook on nursing home management, the scope of the book is much broader.   The conventional text is not likely to include chapters on environmental adaptations, companion animals, families as clients, intergenerational programs, care of the dying and guidelines for a nondiscriminatory application form, as this book does. Several of the chapters include recommended resources for various types of programs in addition to references.

121.   Infeld, Donna L. and John R. Kress (Eds.).   (1989). Cases In Long Term Care: Building the Continuum. Owings Mills, MD: National Health Publishing, 291 pages.

The basic purpose of this book is to provide material for a case study approach that touches briefly on the importance of management In long term care.   The book includes 14 cases organized under the headings of Leadership and Management Decision-Making, Operations, Financial Planning, and Strategic Planning and Community Relations.   Each case describes a facility, presents an issue requiring management decision-making, and offers a resolution as a basis for further discussion.

122.   May, Maurice I., Edvrdas Daminskas and Jack Dasten with David A. Levine. (1991). Managing Institutional Long Term Care for the Elderly. Gaithersburg, MD: Aspen Publishers, 321 pages.

After setting forth the responsibilities of the long term care administrator in terms of six challenges, topics covered include patterns of (resident) care; building an organization; family ties; mental health issues; financial, legal, medical and ethical issues; and marketing, public relations and community involvement. Although addressed primarily to issues of management in large institutions, this volume could be used by both entry-level and experienced administrators.   Appendices containing case examples of functional assessment, examples of job descriptions, policy statements and forms add to its utility.

123.   Moore, Robert and Joan C. Worthem. (1992). "Market and Financial Planning in Senior Care." Topics in Health Care Financing, 18(3):72-79.

The size of the aging population has sparked interest in the senior health care market. However, demographic trends alone are not sufficient to guarantee successful operation of a new facility. This chapter outlines key factors in the success of a venture: an understanding of such market considerations as specialty care, potential clients, potential competition and obtaining a certificate of need. It also addresses financial issues that must be resolved before a venture is undertaken, including deciding whether to develop or to acquire a facility, funding sources, estimating construction costs, pre-occupancy marketing costs and anticipated revenue sources, operating expenses and cash flow.

124.   NAB Study Guide: How to Prepare for the Nursing Home Administrators Examination, Second Edition.   (1992). Washington, DC: National Association of Boards of Examiners for Nursing Home Administrators, Inc., 210 pages.

This study guide is eminently readable and quite adequate for the task it was designed to perform. The bulk of the guide is made up of six chapters by well-known authorities in the domains of practice in which administrators are engaged: patient care; personnel management; financial management; marketing and public relations; physical resource management; and laws, regulatory codes and governing boards. It is a valuable resource for those interested in taking on or understanding the role of the nursing home administrator.

125.   Priest, Stephen L. (1989). Understanding Computer Resources: A Health Care Perspective. Owings Mills, MD: National Health Publishing, 303 pages.

Although not addressed specifically to the use of computers in nursing homes, this book covers many topics that are immediately applicable to them. They range from identifying needs and planning for computer resources (including their acquisition) to ongoing computer resource management.

126.   Shore, Herbert. (1987). "Surviving as an Administrator." Contemporary Long Term Care, 10(10):38-41.

After 36 years as a nursing home administrator, the author discusses the many roles an administrator must play, the groups with which it is necessary to interact, and some personal frustrations and satisfactions. The sections on residents and their families and on the philosophy of working with older persons with impairments are especially valuable.

127.   Toner, John A., Lynn M. Tepper and Beverly Greenfield. (1993). Long Term Care: Management Scope and Practical Issues. Philadelphia, PA: The Charles Press, Publishers, Inc., 230 pages.

This collection of essays, which covers the evolution of long term care, the long-term-care process, problem-solving, ethical considerations and recent mental health legislation on long term care, highlights specific issues in nursing home administration.

Funding

128.   Gertler, Paul J. (1989). "Subsidies, Quality and the Regulation of Nursing Homes." Journal of Public Economics, 38(1):33-52.

The author of this article investigated the effects that Medicaid has in the quality of care received by Medicaid recipients living in nursing homes. It is argued that the Medicaid program cannot at the same time increase access to nursing homes, raise reimbursement payments and increase quality.

129.   Jenkins, Robert K. (1993). "Fund-Raising through Grants." Nursing Homes, 25-27, April.

Topics and sources of funding are outlined for administrators. Steps for preparing grants and information for evaluating programs are given.

130.   Horowitz, Judith L. and Margo P. Kelly. (1991). "Financing Retirement Communities: The Changing Picture." Topics in Health Care Financing, 17(4):49-61.

Financing vehicles for capital development of retirement communities are discussed, including tax-exempt bonds, taxable bonds and commercial loans. An analysis is provided of the types of bonds most appropriate for various operations and the restrictions placed upon such financing by the 1988 Tax Act. Commercial loans are expected to become increasingly important as legislative support for tax-exempt debt fades. Financing of operations is possible through nonrefundable entrance fees, monthly maintenance fees or a combination of both. Methods to project fill-up and turnover, health care utilization, estimates of operating expenses and cash flow are outlined. Questions of hospital investment in continuing care retirement communities (CCRCs) are discussed.

131.   Somers, Anne R.   (1987).   "Insurance for Long Term Care." The New England Journal of Medicine, 317(1):23-29.

This article reasons that a consensus on goals and definition of both health care policy and health care financing policy must precede further legislation. The importance of a continuum of care is discussed. Obstacles to effective reform of long term care are outlined: uncertain public need, heterogeneous populations, complex organizational and administrative problems, technological specialization, concern over uninsurable risk populations and financial exposure. Long term care policy should promote and encompass preventive efforts rather than life extension or prolongation efforts.   The conclusion offers a proposal for guidelines on a national long term care policy.

5

Noninstitutional Care

Alternatives to Institutionalization

132.   Chappell, Neena L. (1991). "Living Arrangements and Sources of Caregiving." Journal of Gerontology, 46(1):S1-8.

The living arrangements of elderly individuals and their possible caregivers are reviewed. The study examines whether proximity determines the type of support provided. Friends were found to be more important for overall support than originally thought. The structural arrangement of living with someone was determined to be the most important factor in receiving assistance with IADL.

133.   Namazi, Kevan H., J. Kevin Eckert, Eva Kahana and Stephanie M. Lyon, editors. (1989). "Psychological well-being of Elderly Board and Care Home Residents." The Gerontologist, 29(4):511-516.

Investigators explored the positive and negative aspects of living arrangements that are less restrictive alternatives to institutions, arrangements such as adult foster care, domiciliary care, or personal care homes. These types of alternatives were seen to be beneficial to discharged patients and older adults without family, and were generally successful in keeping older people out of restrictive facilities while at the same time providing them with a home-like environment.

134.   Powers, James S. (1989). "Helping Family and Patients Decide between Home Care and Nursing Home Care." Southern Medical Journal, 82(6):723-726.

Deciding between home care and nursing home care is difficult for family, patient and physician. Major criteria for making the decision include medical appropriateness, cost, family resources and functional status. One of the most important considerations is the cost of the two types of care. The average cost of one year in a nursing home is over $20,000. Home care may be even higher. However, the actual cost will depend on the complexity of the care and the number of services needed.

135.   Quinn, Joan L. (1987). "Home Health Care" in The Encyclopedia of Aging , George L. Maddox , editor-in-chief. New York, NY: Springer Publishing Co., Inc.

This article presents an overview of home health care, identifying the purposes of home care services and describing four types of home health care organizations, the services available, and qualification and reimbursement sources. A typical user profile is described and a brief historical perspective of the origination of home health care is given. Finally, demonstration projects are mentioned with recommendations for future home health care systems.

136.   Sherwood, Sylvia, David S. Greer, John N. Morris, Vincent Mor and Associates. (1981). An Alternative to Institutionalization: The Highland Heights Experiment. Cambridge, MA: Ballinger Publishing Co., 323 pages.

Highland Heights Apartments for the Physically Impaired and Elderly in Fall River, MA, a medically-oriented apartment complex was the focus of this study. Its architecture, outpatient clinic and other services were shown to have enhanced residents' functioning and offer an alternative to an institution.

137.   Standards and Guidelines for Adult Day Care. (1990). Prepared by the National Institute on Adult Day Care, 224 pages.

The move toward increased professionalism has significantly changed adult day care. The 1990 standards outlined in this publication reflect the recognition of adult day care as a quality service within the continuum of long term care. Guidelines and program profiles are included for dealing with specific patient populations.

Family Caregiving

138.   Gallagher, Dolores (1987). "Caregivers of Chronically Ill Elders" in Encyclopedia of Aging , George L. Maddox, editor-in-chief. New York, NY: Springer Publishing Co., Inc.

Acknowledging the growing recognition that stresses inherent in the caregiving role may often create health problems or mental anguish for the caregiver, this article discusses intervention techniques for decreasing caregiver stress and increasing adaptive coping skills workshops, support groups, psychotherapy, behavioral training, and respite programs. The article concludes that although intervention programs elicit positive response from caregivers, more controlled research is needed, especially to expand the available information, primarily based on Alzheimer's caregiver research, to include caregivers in other areas,

139.   Cantor, Marjorie H. (1991).   "Family and Community: Changing Roles in an Aging Society."   The Gerontologist, 31(3):337-346.

The author contends that the concept of social care is much broader than the provision of formal social services. Such care encompasses both formal and informal services and is best explained by use of a system model which emphasizes the system's interactive and dynamic nature from both individual and ecological perspectives. Primary components of the model, as well as the effects of emerging societal trends on the social care system, are discussed. These include an aging population, family structure and caregiving responsibilities, and integration of the formal and informal care systems. It is within this framework that the author suggests several research questions and policy issues for future study.

140.   Cicirelli, Victor G. (1990). Ethical Beliefs and Elderly Parents' Exercise of Autonomy in Informal Family Caregiving Situations. Washington, DC: AARP Andrus Foundation, 102 pages.

The primary purpose of this monograph was to study the relationship between mothers' and daughters' beliefs in autonomy and paternalism and their impact on decisions regarding family caregiving. In-person interviews were conducted with 50 mother-daughter pairs in which daughters provided 31-42 hours of care weekly. The ANOVA analysis indicated that: a) when both mother and daughter scored high on paternalistic beliefs, paternalistic decisions regarding caregiving were most frequently made and least frequently made when pairs scored low on paternalistic beliefs; b) difference in beliefs between mothers and daughters resulted in greater conflict surrounding caregiving decisions; and c) the more mothers and daughters shared beliefs in autonomy the more often autonomous decisions regarding caregiving were made.

141.   Dayton-Ingersoll, Berit, Nancy Chapman and Margaret Neal. (1990). "A Program for Caregivers in the Workplace." The Gerontologist, 30(1):126-130.

This article describes a program designed to provide support in the workplace for employed caregivers of older relatives. Findings from a preliminary survey of employee views in 33 companies formed the basis for developing a seven-week educational series and service option program (i.e., care planning, support groups, a buddy system) at four demonstration sites. Of the 9,573 survey respondents, almost one-quarter indicated they provided care to older persons. A total of 256 employees or 3% of those who had identified themselves as caregivers attended the seminars; one-third of these were anticipatory caregivers. Data show that the actual percentage of caregivers attending the seminars and participating in the service options was small. The authors propose several recommendations for practice and research.

142. George, Linda K. and Deborah T. Gold. (1990). Easing Caregiver Burden: An Intervention to Overcome Barriers to Service Utilization. Durham, NC: Center for the Study of Aging and Human Development, Duke University Medical Center, 67 pages.

This study developed, tested and evaluated an intervention designed to help caregivers overcome obstacles to use of formal community services, mobilize informal assistance and implement effective coping strategies. The project sample consisted of 264 caregivers of older adults in early stages of dementia. Evaluation data included: a baseline interview performed prior to intervention and three follow-up assessments at six-month intervals to determine to what extent caregivers complied with recommendations made by the study's social workers. Levels of compliance were uniformly high, with caregivers being most successful in implementing recommendations for personal coping strategies. Caregiver "overload" and "burden" were associated with lower levels of compliance; satisfaction with instrumental assistance from friends and families predicted subsequent levels of compliance.

143.   Heath, Angela.   (1993).   Long Distance Caregiving: A
Survival Guide for Far Away Caregivers.   Lakewood, CO:
American Source Books, 122 pages.

This book provides practical, specific information and a
step-by-step planning process for developing an effective,
manageable long distance care plan for family members. This
can help to relieve the frustration, confusion and stress felt by
persons attempting to care for family members across the miles.

144.   Johnson, Colleen L. and Lillian Troll. (1992). "Family
Functioning in Late Life." Journal of Gerontology, 47(2):S66-72.

The focus of this research study was on investigating the breadth
of family support for the oldest old. Data on 150 persons aged 85
years and older (mean age of respondents was 89 years) were
collected and analyzed. Only 5% of the sample had surviving
relatives and slightly less than one-quarter had no available family
resources. However, 35% of the sample reported availability of
a caregiver if needed.   Children provided assistance with
expressive needs but few served as a confidant to their parents.
The use of formal supports did not vary significantly among
different family configurations. Characteristics of family structure
and integration as well as a topology of family resources are
presented in graphic form.

145.   Kosberg, Jordan I., Richard E. Cairl and Donald M. Keller.
(1990). "Components of Burden: Interventive Implications." The
Gerontologist, 30(2):236-242.

The Cost of Care Index (CCI), a multidimensional measure of
caregiving burden, was used to determine the experienced or
anticipated impact of caring for an older relative with Alzheimer's
disease.   The study sample was comprised of 127 informal
caregivers of Alzheimer's disease patients in Florida's Tampa Bay
area.   A series of predictor variables were classified into six
categories, including caregiver characteristics, formal support,

informal support, functioning and consequences, as well as patient functioning. Study results of analyzing overall CCI scores for respondents indicated that burden is significantly related to being female, caring for a patient who exhibits behavior problems and self-reported mental health problems. The author advocates for the use of burden measures for caregivers to assist practitioners in the early identification and intervention of potential caregiving problems.

146.   Krach, Peg. (1991). "Filial Responsibility and Financial Strain: The Impact on Farm Families." Journal of Gerontological Nursing, 16(7):38-41.

The purpose of the study was to investigate how rural adults perceive their filial responsibility and affection for their aged parents the extent to which financial strain adult children affects that perception. The sample was comprised of 296 farmers over the age of 45 who had at least one living parent over the age of 65 who was not residing in the same house. Lower levels of affection were found among subjects who were financially strained, but financial concerns did not appear to affect filial responsibility.

147.   Linsk, Nathan L., Sharon M. Keigher and Suzanne E. England. (1992). Wages for Caring: Compensating Family Care of the Elderly. New York, NY: Praeger, 281 pages.

The central theme of this book is that family caregivers are often overlooked in the framing of formal home care programs. It is pointed out that joint partnerships are possible and often preferred by consumers. Part One describes the responsibilities involved in caring for an older person and existing public policies and introduces the issue of compensating a family for caring for a relative. Part Two evaluates programs that have been implemented on a trial basis. Part Three discusses the impact of providing financial support for long term care.

148.   Penning, Margaret J. (1990). "Receipt of Assistance by
Elderly People: Hierarchical Selection and Task Specificity." The
Gerontologist, 30(2):220-227.

This article presents research on two models of informal social
and behavioral support for older persons: the hierarchical
compensatory model and the task specificity model. A stratified
random sample of 1,284 non-institutionalized persons 60 years
of age and older living in Winnipeg, Manitoba, Canada comprised
the study sample. Among measures included in the data analysis
were types and sources of assistance received, measures of
availability of social support as well as age, gender, education and
health status.

149.   Rubinstein, Robert L., Baine B. Alexander, Marene M.
Goodman and Mark Luborsky. (1991). "Key Relationships of
Never Married, Childless Older Women: A Cultural Analysis."
Journal of Gerontology: Social Sciences, 46(5):S270-277.

This article explores the key relationships of childless older
women. Qualitative research conversations were held with 31
never married, childless women aged 60 and older. The authors
report on the types, attitudes and limits of key personal
relationships of these women as well as describe strategies they
have employed to develop "kin-like" relationships and to solve
problems concerning expectations of care in later life.

150.   Sherman, Susan R. and Evelyn S. Newman. (1988).
Foster Families For Adults. New York, NY: Columbia University
Press, 318 pages.

One option for care of older persons that has received limited
discussion is foster family care. This book explores this option
within a continuum of sheltered housing for adults, and focuses
specifically on the integration of the resident into the host family
and into the larger community. Also explored are the roles of the
foster family, the resident and agency personnel.

151.   Stone, Robin I. and Peter Kemper. (1989). "Spouses and Children of Disabled Elders: How Large a Constituency for Long Term Care Reform?" The Milbank Quarterly, 67(34):485-506.

A wealth of current demographic information on the numbers of potential and active caregivers of chronically disabled older persons is presented. Statistical estimates are extrapolated from the 1984 National Long Term Care Survey and applied to U.S. Census Bureau figures. The authors caution that although the extent of emotional, financial and physical support provided caregivers should not be underestimated, the numbers of children and spouses who provide care of older persons as well as child care or employment responsibilities are relatively small. The future impact of shifts in the availability of informal caregivers on public policy agendas for the older population is discussed.

152.   White-Means, Shelly I. and Michael C. Thornton. (1990). "Labor Market Choices and Home Health Care Provision among Employed Ethnic Caregivers." The Gerontologist, 30(6):769-775.

This paper analyzes the differences and similarities in the decisions racial/ethnic caregivers make regarding the number of hours allocated to care and the labor market. Results indicate there are significant differences between ethnic groups regarding caregiving hours and employment decisions. When greater ADL limitations among care recipients result in loss of labor hours for the caregiver, women are more likely to cut back on employment to provide care. Afro-Americans are more likely to provide more care hours than are white ethnics. If the caregiver lives with the care recipient fewer hours of informal care are provided, and caregivers without substitutes provide the most caregiving hours. Implications of findings for policy and future research are discussed.

Homebound Elderly

153.   Edelman, Perry and Susan L. Hughes. (1990). "The Impact of Community Care on Provision of Informal Care to Homebound Elderly Persons." Journal of Gerontology: Social Sciences, 45(2):S74-84.

This study examines the relationship between the number and level of formal and informal services provided to homebound older persons at nine and 48 months after the initiation of formal care. The original study sample was comprised of 157 clients of the Five Hospital Program (a Chicago-based long term home care program for chronically ill homebound elderly) and 156 clients of home-delivered meal programs in the same geographical area. Of those clients remaining in the study, 91% at nine months and 68% at 48 months were receiving community care. Study findings imply that supplementation of informal services by formal community care occurred significantly more frequently than either substitution or specialization/reallocation. There was a significant increase in the extent of formal services provided to both groups of clients at nine months and to community care clients at 48 months.   Multivariate regression analyses found only limited impact of community care on formal care. Overall, it appears that informal caregivers continue to assist homebound older people over time, even after the introduction of formal services.

154.   Folden, Susan L. (1990). "On the Inside Looking Out: Perceptions of the Homebound." Journal of Gerontological Nursing, 16(1):9-15.

Ethnographic methods were used to explore seven chronically ill older adults' perspectives on being homebound. Findings suggest that older homebound adults are acutely aware and affected by losses in their life and are especially vulnerable to concurrent losses. Specific losses of most concern to respondents were loss of independence, social networks, financial independence and personal control over their lives. However, being homebound was not expressly identified as a negative consequence of their illness and respondents reported they had made as many changes as possible to modify their environments so they could be as independent as possible.

155.   Hereford, Russell W. (1989). "Developing Nontraditional Home-Based Services for the Elderly." Quality Review Bulletin, 15(3):92-97, March.

In May 1986 the Robert Wood Johnson Foundation initiated the Supportive Services Program for Older Persons, designed to supplement traditional home health care services with additional needed non-medical services on a fee-for-service basis. Based on previous research findings, the following services package was offered: house-based services (specifically physical environment maintenance), case management and related services and special services (such as personal emergency response systems, health screening and home-delivered groceries/drugs, etc.). First-year program evaluation findings verified the existence of a private market among primarily well older consumers.

156.   Pelham, Anabel O. and William F. Clark (Eds.). (1986). Managing Home Care for the Elderly: Lessons from Community-Based Agencies. New York, NY: Springer Publishing Co., Springer Series on Adulthood and Aging, Volume 15, 196 pages.

This book is a collection of essays concerning projects funded by HCFA to maintain frail older persons in their homes. The editors consider community-based long term care services to be "institutions." The struggles of organizations to serve as both family and formal organizations are chronicled.

157.   Wister, Andrew.   (1992).   "Residential Attitudes and Knowledge: Use and Future Use of Home Support Agencies." The Journal of Applied Gerontology, 11(1):84-100.

This article examines health beliefs and attitude measures as integral components of health service. Data analysis is based on interview responses from 280 persons aged 74 years and older residing in Ontario, Canada. Major study findings were: 1) greater emphasis on independence and self-reliance conform with higher levels of service knowledge; 2) users of in-home programs tend to be knowledgeable about the services, live alone and perceive a greater health need; and 3) anticipated future use of in-home services was greater for respondents living alone and those with deteriorating functional ability. The author concludes with a discussion of findings in terms of their relevance for service providers and policy makers.

6

Housing

Housing Alternatives

158.   Golant, Stephen M. (1992). <u>Housing America's Elderly:
Many Possibilities, Few Choices</u>.   Newbury Park, CA: Sage
Publications, 354 pages.

Public policy questions concerning housing for the elderly are
addressed in this book. Topics include problems with conventional
dwellings, planned age-segregated housing, rent-subsidized
housing, care to facilitate aging in place, group housing,
retirement facilities, and questions surrounding land use and Fair
Housing Act restrictions.

159.   Newcomer, Robert J., M. Powell Lawton and Thomas O.
Byerts (Eds.).   (1986).   <u>Housing an Aging Society: Issues,
Alternatives and Policy</u>. New York, NY: Van Nostrand Reinhold,
246 pages.

This anthology looks at two trends: the widening of the range of
housing alternatives that have developed as a component of the
system of care for older adults and the growing need for
specialists in the health and social service fields to better

understand the use of different housing forms in light of current
social realities and social programs.

160.   Regnier, Victor and Jon Pynoos (Eds.). (1987). Housing
the Aged: Design Directives and Policy Considerations. New
York, NY: Elsevier Science Publishing, 500 pages.

This book synthesizes the often disparate fields of housing design
for older persons and public policy considerations concerning
housing for older persons. It is designed to sensitize sponsors,
designers, planners, developers and managers to the
characteristics and needs of the end users of their product and
shows how the living environments they create can be improved.
In separate sections, it looks at design for the well older person,
supportive housing for persons who are moderately impaired, and
housing environments for the frail older person.

161.   Strategies for Senior Housing Underwriting-Evaluating
Senior Housing Developments.   (1990).   Mortgage Bankers
Association of America, 152 pages.

The purpose of this book is to evaluate trends for senior citizen
housing and to discuss the ability to meet their needs.   The
industry is discussed in detail, especially approaches to
developing a successful retirement community.

Aging in Place

162.   Boles, Daralia D. (1989). "Aging in Place in the 1990s."
Progressive Architecture, 84-92, November.

The concept of assisted living has expanded the options available
to older persons as total life care has become more accepted. A
continuum of care ranges from independent living through
assisted living to skilled nursing. This article looks at how building

design can enhance the life care experience for residents of facilities that provide it.

163.   Cullinane, Patrick. (1992). "Neighborhoods That Make Sense: Community Allies for Elders Aging in Place." Generations, 69-72, Spring.

Older persons who wish to "age in place" not only need a formal system to allow them to do this safely, but also an understanding by individuals in the community and neighborhood as to what this population needs.   With the help of the community, the neighborhood can act as an alternative to institutional care. There is a need for older persons to go beyond the traditional aging network and form alliances with organizations and businesses that have not traditionally addressed their needs. Several programs that seek to link older persons to a nontraditional network are identified in this article.

164.   Dibner, Andrew S. (Ed.). (1992). Personal Response Systems: An International Report of a New Home Care Service. New York, NY: The Haworth Press, Inc., 249 pages.

A review of international emergency response system technology is presented in this book. Information is provided about service demand and provision, economics and financing, operational issues, demographics and the integration of personal response systems into health care systems. The editor speaks to the psychological effects of an emergency response system upon older persons and caregivers, and implications of the system for both groups.

165.   Koncelik, Joseph A. (1982).   Aging and the Product Environment. Stroudsburg, PA: Hutchinson Ross Publishing Co., 200 pages.

Industrial design as it affects older persons is the focus of this book. The author looked at how the aging process impacts the need for designs that differ from standard ones, and then examined living environments, furnishings, and appliances and automobiles from the perspective of being old.

166.   Reschovsky, James D. and Sandra J. Newman. (1990). "Adaptations for Independent Living by Older Frail Households." The Gerontologist, 30(4):543-552.

This study explored three categories of adaptation activities that frail householders undertake to remain independent and maintain normal functioning in a community-based household. These include home operation activities, housing consumption adjustments and health-related activities. A statistical analysis was based on the Survey of Housing Adjustments (SHA) conducted by the U.S. Census Bureau as a supplement to the 1979 Houston, Texas Standard Metropolitan Statistical Area (SMSA) Annual Housing Survey of households where the head of house or spouse was 55 or older. The sample was comprised of 1,070 households. The authors found that frail members of households appeared to behave no differently than the non-frail in addressing home repair and maintenance needs. About 40% of those with mobility limitations reported at least one housing modification that was needed and was lacking. The residents who were the most vulnerable and frail had low incomes, rental status and lacked informal support either within or outside the household.

167.   Rowles, Graham D. (1993). "Evolving Images of Place in Aging and 'Aging in Place.'" Generations, 17(2):65-70.

Humans have a propensity to develop an affinity for the physical places in which they live. The concept of aging in place has deep roots in American culture. As home-ownership has become an important goal of American society, aging in place has become even more important. However, accommodating aging in place has failed to be made a part of social policy. Policymakers have tended to encourage the placement of the elderly in special environments such as retirement housing units and nursing homes. In 1939 the U.S. Census counted 1,200 nursing homes with 25,000 beds. By 1960, there had been increases to 9,582 nursing homes with 331,000 beds. In 1970 the count was 23,000 homes with over a million residents. During this time the concept of the nursing home as a normative final place of residence began to emerge, thus reinforcing the concept of old age as a time of relocation. The author points out that public policymakers have only recently begun to recognize the value of aging in place.

168.   Tilson, David (Ed.). (1990). <u>Aging in Place: Supporting the Frail Elderly in Residential Environments</u>. Glenview, IL: Scott, Foresman and Co., 315 pages.

This compilation contains essays by leading researchers on the question of aging in place. It discusses the dimensions of the current trend toward encouraging institutionalization rather than allowing older persons to age in place. It looks at current residential possibilities including independent living, congregate housing, residential care facilities and continuing care retirement communities. It discusses the public policy setting that surrounds aging in place and concludes with a look ahead at questions about this issue that will need to be answered.

Continuing Care Retirement Communities

169.   Armeill, Bruce P. (1984). "Private Hilltop Village Offers Residents Every Amenity of Home." <u>Hospitals</u>, <u>58</u>(4):90 and 92.

Duncaster, a upper-income, private, not-for-profit, 300-person life care community hilltop village in Bloomfield, CT is described. Duncaster's older residents live in three neighborhoods that radiate from a central village. Community facilities surround an open town green.

170.   Carstens, Diane Y. (1985). Site Planning and Design for the Elderly: Issues, Guidelines and Alternatives. New York, NY: Van Nostrand Reinhold, 170 pages.

The issues and suggestions presented in this book are focused on one facet of design: outdoor spaces surrounding planned housing developments for well older persons. The book is written to sensitize designers to the functional, perceptual and social changes that come with the aging process, as well as to outline recommendations for spatial organization and design of outdoor spaces.

171.   Cohen, Marc A. et al. (1989). "Patterns of Nursing Home Use in the Prepaid Managed Care System: The Continuing Care Retirement Community." The Gerontologist, 29(1):74-78.

The purpose of this study was to analyze the use of nursing home services in continuing care retirement communities (CCRCs) compared with their use in the general community. Residents of these CCRCs appear to use nursing homes more often for short-term, recuperative care than do residents of the general community use nursing homes for that purpose. There is evidence that CCRC managers respond to the financial incentives inherent in prepaid long term care by using the nursing home more cost effectively.

172.   Lumpkin, James R. (1990). Retirement Housing and Long Term Health Care Choice of the Elderly. Washington, DC: AARP Andrus Foundation, 70 pages.

This study was designed to evaluate the way older consumers conduct the long term health care service decision process. The majority of a national sample consisted of older adults who were living independently in the community as well as a small proportion (5%) who were residents of retirement facilities. The findings suggested that: 1) most respondents (44%) began considering and searching for a retirement facility between the ages of 70 and 79; 2) although asking and receiving advice from others, older respondents visited potential facilities and made the relocation decision on their own; 3) safety features were rated as the most important attribute of a retirement and/or long term care facility; 4) overall, respondents had negative attitudes toward nursing homes (objecting to the structure of the environment and lack of privacy) and viewed them as a place of last resort; and 5) a majority of the older respondents would prefer to have both retirement and long term care facilities at the same location.

173.   Stearns, Lisa R. et al.   (1990).   "Lessons from the Implementation of CCRC Regulation."   The Gerontologist, 30(2):154-161.

Efficient regulation of CCRCs depends on appropriate legislation and adequate implementation of the law, as well as regulations to protect both residents who pay large endowments and residents who pay on a fee-for-service basis. This article looks at what lessons have been learned to date and what needs to be addressed in future public policy.

7

Costs of Long Term Care

174.   Branch, Laurence G. et al. (1988). "Impoverishing the Elderly: A Case Study of the Financial Risk of Spend-Down among Massachusetts Elderly People."   The Gerontologist, 28(5):648-652.

This study estimates the risk of impoverishment resulting from the cost of institutional or home-based care, in spite of Medicaid's protective measures. If admitted to a skilled nursing facility, half of the older persons living alone would spend to impoverishment in 13 weeks. Of couples, one of whom is admitted to a long term care facility, 25% spend to impoverishment in 13 weeks, and over half within one year.

175.   Coburn, Andrew F. et al. (1993). "Effect of Prospective Reimbursement on Nursing Home Costs." HRS: Health Service Research, 28(1):45-68.

In July of 1982, the State of Maine implemented a prospective payment system to control Medicaid costs.   Prospective reimbursement limits Medicaid payments to nursing homes to rates set in advance, regardless of actual costs incurred. The authors of this article sought to determine how well costs were controlled by this action. Findings indicated a decline in the rate of growth in nursing home costs in the two years following implementation of prospective reimbursement. The most efficiency appears to have been produced in the areas of room and board costs. However, by the third year after implementation, responsiveness to the financial incentives appears to have declined, with fewer facilities achieving savings and more breaking even or incurring losses. Some evidence also exists that the system may have reduced the quality of care and access to Medicaid care.

176.   Ehreth, Jennifer. (1992). "Cost Methodology in Long Term Care Evaluations." Medical Care Review, 49(3):331-353.

Methods associated with assessing costs of long term care have received little attention in the literature. This article synthesizes the literature on long term care cost methodology, discusses cost accounting and economic applications to long term care and presents a framework for evaluating the costs associated with long term care services. A conceptual model is introduced that is designed to measure and predict two levels of cost: program (micro) and system (macro).

177.   Kolb, Deborah S., Peter J. Veysey and Joseph L. Gocke. (1991). "Private Long Term Care Insurance: Will it Work?" Topics in Health Care Financing, 17(4):9-21.

Currently, Medicaid pays 44% of all long term care costs, individuals pay 48%, and private insurance pays about 1%. The need for reforming the system has focused attention on private long term care insurance. At first glance, private long term care insurance has a great deal of appeal. It is a privately-financed solution that would require no federal money and has the potential to reach a great many Americans. Despite these advantages, the authors predict that private long term care insurance will not become a leading mechanism for financing long term care in the future. Problems with it include costs which are too high for most older persons, difficulty in projecting what typical long term care costs will be in the future, and uncertainty about future legislation and tax considerations. Despite efforts by the National Association of Insurance Commissioners and other groups to educate the public and politicians on the need for insurance, members of the "baby boom" generation have been more concerned with their immediate needs. Providers should not expect them to have a significant impact on demand or payment of long term care services for at least 10 years.

178.   Liu, Korbin, Maria Perokek and Kenneth Manton. (1993). "Catastrophic Acute and Long Term Care Costs: Risks Faced by Disabled Elderly Persons." The Gerontologist, 33(3):229-307.

The major reasons for the repeal of the Medicare Catastrophic Coverage Act are discussed, noting that the most significant omission was a long term care benefit. There is an analysis of the extent to which a need for acute and long term care cause older persons with disabilities to incur catastrophic costs. It was found that when costs of long term care were included, the out-of-pocket costs for older persons with disabilities rose to a level considered catastrophic.

179.   Rivlin, Alice M. and Joshua M. Wiener. (1988). Caring for the Disabled Elderly: Who Will Pay? Washington, DC: The Brookings Institution, 318 pages.

This study analyzes the major options for reforming the way long term care is financed. It first looks at the potential market for private long term care insurance and other private sector initiatives. Then it reviews various public sector programs and their advantages and disadvantages. It recommends both a greatly expanded role for the private sector in financing long term care and a new public insurance program.

180.   Wiener, Joshua M. and Laurel H. Illston.   (1993).
"Options for Long Term Care Financing Reform: Public and
Private Insurance Strategies." The Journal of Long Term Care
Administration, 21(4):46-57.

The debate over reforming long term care financing is primarily
a debate over the roles of the private and public sectors. These
authors propose that, when examining the two alternatives, five
concepts should be considered: recognizing long term care as a
normal risk of aging, the need to protect the older persons from
financial ruin, preventing dependence on welfare, recognizing that
institutionalization is not always the best alternative and the need
to improve quality of care. Since only 10-20% of older persons
can afford private long term care insurance, several ways to make
it more affordable have been proposed: encouraging purchase of
long term care insurance when young, tax incentives for
purchasing a policy and easier access to Medicaid for those who
purchase a state-approved policy.

8

Minorities

181.   Choi, Namkee G.   (1991).   "Racial Differences in the Determinants of Living Arrangements of Widowed and Divorced Elderly Women."   The Gerontologist, 31(4):496-497.

This article investigates factors associated with single ethnically diverse older women's decisions regarding living alone or living with others. The primary goal was to examine differences in the determinants of living arrangements within racial groups. Data analysis focused on comparisons of economic and sociodemographic variables on living arrangements of white and nonwhite widows and divorcees. For all widows, results suggest that those who raised more children, were nonwhite, poor and had shorter work histories were less likely to live alone. Nonwhite single women were more likely to live alone than white single women. Poverty status appears to have had little effect on the reasons why nonwhite single women lived alone, with family variables and marital history more significant determinants than economic affordability.

182.   Greene, Ruth L. and Ilene C. Siegler. (1984). "Blacks." In Erdman B. Palmore (Ed.) Handbook on the Aged in the United States. Westport, CT: Greenwood Press, 219-233.

The authors relate how the differences in life experiences between different cohorts of African-Americans have shaped the ways in which their experiences as older people differ from each other and from the general population. They also discuss research issues related to African-American older persons and in what direction they feel future research should go.

183.   Harel, Zev, Edward A. McKinney and Michael Williams (Eds.). (1990). Black Aged: Understanding Diversity and Service Needs. Newbury Park, CA: Sage Publications, 264 pages.

This volume looks at the unique life-styles and circumstances of the older African-American in the United States. It also examines service needs and how those needs are being met or not being met.

184.   Jackson, James S., Linda M. Chatters and Robert J. Taylor. (1993). Aging in Black America. Newbury Park, CA: Sage Publications, 338 pages.

These authors examine the status and special conditions of older blacks and includes chapters on the African-American community, churches and religion, retirement, health, political participation and other issues.

185.   Kii, Toshi. (1984). "Asians." In Erdman B. Palmore (Ed.) Handbook on the Aged in the United States. Westport, CT: Greenwood Press, 201-217.

This author relates how older Asians differ from the general population of older persons. She also discusses the fallacy that Asian-Americans have the same attitudes about their elders that their counterparts in various countries of origin have. The idea that Asian-Americans take care of their own rather than depending on social service networks is also discussed.

186.   Lacayo, Carmela G. (1984). "Hispanics." In Erdman B. Palmore (Ed.) Handbook on the Aged in the United States. Westport, CT: Greenwood Press, 253-267.

This article describes the growing Hispanic older population in the United States and its underutilization of needed social services. It also describes how differences from the general population in educational level and socioeconomic status have affected this population.

187.   Miranda, Manuel R. (1992). "Minorities and Aging: Studies in Diversity." Perspective on Aging, 21(1):4-10.

The author's expertise and knowledge in the area of public policy issues facing minority elderly is reflected in this review of the magnitude of the problems and possible solutions. Current statistical data from the 1990 U.S. Bureau of the Census present the statistical ethical and racial diversity of our country's older adults specifically in the areas of education, income and assets, living arrangements and access to health care. Recommendations are made for changes in the socio-environmental factors affecting ethnic minority older persons in order to provide a setting for structuring effective public policies.

188.   National Indian Council on Aging. (1984). "Indian and Alaskan Natives." In Erdman B. Palmore (Ed.) Handbook on the Aged in the United States. Westport, CT: Greenwood Press, 269-276.

This chapter discusses the differences in aging patterns between older Indians and the general population. These differences include income, education, employment levels, the importance of the extended family, and physical and mental health problems.

189.   Wallace, Steven P. and Chin-Yin Lew-Ting. (1992). "Getting By at Home: Community-Based Long Term Care of

Latino Elders." Cross-Cultural Medicine A Decade Later (Special Issue). Western Journal of Medicine, 157(3):334-337.

This study compared the health of older Latinos to that of non-Latinos. Over the age of 65, Latinos had lower death rates than whites from most causes, but made more physician visits and had more hospitalization. The Latino culture is discussed in relationship to the use of health care. The findings indicate the need for physician referral to in-home health services when an older patient is physically disabled.

190.   Worobey, Jacqueline L. and Ronald J. Angel. (1990). "Poverty and Health: Older Minority Women and the Rise of the Female-Headed Household." Journal of Health and Social Behavior, 31:370-383.

This study examines the relationship between poverty and health and the impact of these factors on the establishment of female-headed households among black, Hispanic and white older women. The study sample was comprised of 8,514 black, Hispanic and white women aged 55 to 90 selected from respondents to the 1984 National Health Interview Survey, Supplement on Aging. Findings suggest that black and Hispanic women are more likely to form multigenerational households because of economic need than are white older women. However, poor health was shown to be a major determinant of the decision to live with others.

9

Special Population Groups

191.   Calkins, Margaret P.   (1988).   <u>Design for Dementia:
Planning Environments for the Elderly and Confused</u>. Owings
Mills, MD: National Health Publishing, 151 pages.

This book grew out of a Master of Architecture thesis and is a
practical primer on how dementia units can be designed to
enhance patient experiences. The first section discusses issues
surrounding dementia care and the second section is a guide to
designing specifically for dementia patients.

192.   Cameron, Daniel J. et al. (1987). "Specialized Dementia
Unit: Cost and Benefit Analysis." <u>New York Medical Quarterly</u>,
<u>7</u>:103-107.

This journal article presents a cost, benefit and reimbursement
analysis of a specialized 46-bed dementia unit. The unit was
opened in October 1984 within an academically-affiliated skilled
nursing facility. The findings suggest that nursing homes should
consider forming specialized dementia units and that health care
planners should modify payment systems to support such
endeavors.

193.   Clemmer, William, M.   (1993).   <u>Victims of Dementia Services, Support and Care</u>.   New York, NY: The Hayworth Pastoral Press, 161 pages.

This book relates the history of an early unit for the cognitively disabled and memory impaired. Those working with victims of dementia or planning a similar unit will find this an interesting reference.

194.   Cohen, Uriel and Gerald D. Weisman.   (1991).   <u>Holding on to Home: Designing Environments for People with Dementia</u>. Baltimore, MD: Johns Hopkins University Press, 181 pages.

This book seeks to expand the reader's view of the potential influence of architectural settings on the lives of persons with dementia and to suggest flexible ideas and generalizable directions for improving those settings. It gives principles for the planning and design of facilities for persons with dementia and shows five prototypical facilities that illustrate those principles. The concluding chapter discusses the evaluation of environments for persons with dementia.

195.   Congress of the United States, Office of Technology Assessment.   (1992).   <u>Special Care Units for People with Alzheimer's and Other Dementias: Consumer Education, Research, Regulatory and Reimbursement Issues</u> (Summary). Washington, DC: U.S. Government Printing Office, 56 pages.

This report discusses policy implications for special care units, as well as policy implications, legal and ethical issues, alternatives to special care units, and the nursing home reform provisions of OBRA-87. It concludes with OTA's assessment of the need for establishment of regulations for special care units.

196.   Conrad, Kendon J. and Rosalie Guttman. (1991). "Characteristics of Alzheimer's versus Non-Alzheimer's Adult Day Care Centers." Research on Aging, 13(1).

Adult day care (ADC) centers are often used as an alternative to nursing homes. This article compares ADC centers where more than 30% of the population have Alzheimer's with centers having few Alzheimer's patients in an effort to determine how programs and Alzheimer's Special Care should adapt to an increasing number of demented patients.

197.   Coons, Dorothy H. and Lena Metzelaar. (1990). Manual for Trainers of Direct Service Staff in Special Dementia Units. Ann Arbor, MI: University of Michigan, 205 pages.

This training manual was designed to prepare staff to work in dementia care units. The sessions described focus on providing care and improved quality of life for patients with cognitive impairment and increasing job satisfaction for special care unit staff members. Training methods utilized include lectures, audiovisuals, discussion sessions, exercises and role-playing, and handouts.

198.   Droste, Therese. (1987). "Interest in Alzheimer's Centers Growing." Hospital, 61(8):112.

This article discusses development of hospital-based Alzheimer's disease centers and explains the advantages and the difficulties of combining skills of many disciplines in this effort. Several hospital-based Alzheimer's disease centers are described.

199.   Fox, Patrick. (1989). "From Senility to Alzheimer's Disease: The Rise of the Alzheimer's Disease Movement." Milbank Quarterly, 67(1):58-101.

The author reviews the various factors associated with the emergence of Alzheimer's disease as a major social and health problem in this country. The review includes the historical context of Alzheimer's disease and senile dementia, and the shift in the biomedical conceptualization of the disease from one associated with cognitive decline and aging to one with specific pathological characteristics and symptoms. A discussion of the social structural conditions within the National Institutes of Health and the newly established National Institute on Aging that facilitated the growth and mobilization of the Alzheimer's disease social movement is presented.

200.   Gibson, John W., Janice Rabkin and Robin Munson. (1992). "Critical Issues in Serving the Developmentally Disabled Elderly." Journal of Gerontological Social Work, 19(1):35-49.

The number of older persons with developmental disabilities is increasing rapidly. This study reports the results of 29 in-depth interviews with key members of the developmentally disabled and aging services networks, The results center on the three most frequently mentioned concerns of service providers: 1) aging and health care, 2) access to community care, and 3) family caregivers and advocates. It is suggested that service providers will be unable to meet the burgeoning needs of the number of older persons with developmental disabilities.

201.   Gold, Deborah T. et al. (1991). "Special Care Units: A Typology of Care Settings for Memory-Impaired Older Adults." The Gerontologist, 31(4):467-475.

Special care units (SCUs) are seen by these authors as better settings for memory-impaired older adults because of the concentrated attention on the special needs of the dementia patient. After 55 homes were rated, a typology of care settings was created in this study. SCUs were associated with higher quality of care for patients suffering from dementia, although the care was not consistently high.

202.   Holmes, Douglas et al. (1990). "Impacts Associated with Special Care Units in Long Term Care." Gerontologist, 30(2):178-183.

This journal article discusses a six-month longitudinal study comparing the characteristics of demented patients who were placed in special care units of four nursing homes with those of similar patients in the same nursing homes who were not placed in the special care units.

203.   Koff, Theodore H. (1987). "Nursing Home Management of Alzheimer's Disease: Establishing Standards of Care." Journal of Long Term Care Administration, 15(4):4.

This article recommends establishment of nationwide standards for special nursing home units for Alzheimer's patients. It summarizes recent federal and California legislation related to Alzheimer's, specifies nine criteria for establishing an Alzheimer's program and argues that new standards of care are needed to ensure that Alzheimer's patients and their families can be served with the greatest possible skill and compassion.

204.   Lawton, M. Powell, Mark Fulcomer and Morton H. Kleban. (1984). "Architecture for the Mentally Impaired." Environment and Behavior, 16(6):730-757.

After a post-occupancy evaluation was conducted on the design environment of a nursing facility for residents with mental impairments, comparisons between a traditional and new facility revealed behavioral changes that appeared related to changes made in the environment. Evaluations were based on direct observation of the patients as well as comments of visitors and staff members. The results suggested that increased space, stimulation of environmental awareness, more meaningful activity for the patients, and an increase in visits to patients had positive effects. However, a disadvantage of increased space and privacy was the loss of some social interaction.

205.   Millard, Susan M. (1989). "Maintaining Control of the Alzheimer's Unit." Nursing Homes and Senior Citizen Care, 38(21):13-16.

This article describes the redesign of the Alzheimer's unit at Goodwin House West, a self-contained retirement community in Falls Church, Virginia, which is home to residents both with and without impaired physical and mental abilities. The article describes the residents and staff and the community's physical organization.   Prior to the redesign, Alzheimer's patients frequently wandered away from the unit, entering other residents' rooms and creating a disturbance. The article describes the modifications made to the community which led to an improvement in the atmosphere of the unit and the entire facility.

206.   Morgan, David L. (1989). Caregivers for Elderly Alzheimer's Victims: A Comparison of Caregiving in the Home and in Institutions. Washington, DC: AARP Andrus Foundation, 78 pages.

The purpose of this study was to examine caregiving in formal care settings, as compared to caregiving in the home to better understand the experiences of caregivers of persons with Alzheimer's disease. Special attention was given to the study of factors that affect caregivers' level of involvement and specific burdens associated with caregiving in both settings. The project sample was recruited from the local Alzheimer's Disease Association contact list.   The 191 caregiver respondents completed questionnaires at 18 data collection sites, followed by 31 focus group discussions. Analysis of both quantitative and qualitative data indicated that the level and type of involvement was crucial to understanding the differences between formal and informal caregivers.   The questionnaire data showed that home-based caregivers spent more total hours in their caregiving, but the focus groups showed that formal care caregivers experienced more emotional burden from their involvement.

207.   Namazi, Kevan H. (1991). "A Model Unit: The Corrinne Dolan Alzheimer Center." Nursing Homes and Senior Citizen Care, 40(1).

Many facilities are designed for aesthetic reasons, without features that make caring for Alzheimer's patients easier. This article showcases an Alzheimer's care facility that was designed with the patients and their special needs considered foremost.

208.   Peppard, Nancy R. (1986). "Special Nursing Home Units for Residents with Primary Degenerative Dementia: Alzheimer's Disease." Journal of Gerontology and Social Work, 9(2):5-13.

This article describes a program to develop special units in nursing homes for Alzheimer's patients. The ideal unit is described as having approximately 18 beds, semiprivate rooms, and an active but consistent routine. The residents should be selected after assessment with a dementia scale (the Global Deterioration Scale was used) and should be determined to have non-treatable dementias. Daily activities should be geared to the level of each resident and practiced in groups. The article describes the selection of staff members and their training, and the involvement of patients' families.

209.   Peppard, Nancy R. and Barbara McHugh. (1988). "Staff Sense of Ownership Key to Special Needs Unit Success." Provider, 14(5):30.

This article examines variables that contribute to the successful management of a special needs dementia unit (SNU). The authors explain that SNUs operate under the psychosocial model with a medical component, rather than the medical model traditionally followed by nursing homes. Since a psychosocial model is harder to implement and maintain than a medical model and may have management problems, it is pointed out that a sense of "ownership" and direct involvement in the development and operation of the unit is crucial to its success.

210.   Rabins, Peter V.   (1986).   "Establishing Alzheimer's Disease Units in Nursing Homes: Pros and Cons." Hospital and Community Psychiatry, 37(2):120-121 .

This article examines the issues involved in establishing specialized centers within nursing homes for people with Alzheimer's disease or other cognitive impairments. Pros include recruitment of interested professional staff, concentration of resources, and segregation of impaired residents from the general nursing home population.   Cons include higher resource requirements, the small number of patients that can be treated by such units, and resistance from families and patients who may not think the illness is severe enough for the patient to be kept in such a unit.

211.   Sloane, P. D. and L. J. Mathew (Eds.). (1991). Dementia Units in Long Term Care.   Baltimore, MD: Johns Hopkins University Press.

This book contains 14 chapters that address the topic of special units for dementia patients within nursing homes. A major focus is on a five-state study comparing the characteristics and outcomes of specialized dementia care units with those of non-segregated nursing homes, which showed that special units created an improved quality in at least some facets of living. The book also discusses the design and implementation of special units, the characteristics of residents with dementia, organization and staffing, and planned activities.

212.   Spohr, Betty Baker and Jean Valens Bullard. (1990). To Hold a Falling Star: A Personal Story of Living at Home with Alzheimer's. Stanford, CT: Longmeadow Press, 213 pages.

This is Betty Spohr's powerful story about 12 years of caring for her husband Hank after he was diagnosed with Alzheimer's. It describes with candor the traumas, triumphs and events of living at home with a loved one who has Alzheimer's disease.

213.   Straley, P. F. and K. L. Cameron. (1991). "Operating a Financially Viable Alzheimer's Disease Treatment Unit." Topics in Health Care Financing, 17(4):32-41.

This article describes the specific needs of Alzheimer's disease patients with regard to development of segregated treatment units in hospitals and nursing homes. Four examples of facilities that provide Alzheimer's disease care in special units are provided. Each unit is described in detail and several common characteristics are identified. The article concludes that some changes must be made in financing systems if Alzheimer's disease treatment units of good quality are to continue in operation.

214.   Weiner, Audrey S. and Jacob Reingold. (1989). "Special Care Units for Dementia: Current Practice Models." Journal of Long Term Care Administration, 17(1):14-19.

This article, based on a descriptive national survey, reviews current institutional responses to the care of persons with Alzheimer's disease in nursing home special care units (SCUs). Information is provided on the survey of the environment and activities of SCUs and related programs, and the objectives, environment and nursing staff levels of SCUs.

215.   Welch, H. Gilbert, John S. Walsh and Eric B. Larson. (1992). "The Cost of Institutional Care in Alzheimer's Disease: Nursing Home and Hospital Use in a Prospective Cohort." Journal of the American Geriatrics Society, 40(3).

Society faces a quandary in caring for older Americans with Alzheimer's because of increased demand coupled with limited financial resources. This study looks at 123 patients with Alzheimer's-type dementia, analyzes costs for patients admitted both to hospitals and to nursing homes, and reviews the utility of cost-effectiveness analysis as applied to this problem.

216.   Wiley, Dorothy. (1991). "Success Stories from ARA Special Care Units." <u>Nursing Homes and Senior Citizen Care</u>, <u>40</u>(1).

ARA Living Centers is the largest privately-held provider of long term care. Of its 230 facilities, 34 have special care units called Alzheimer's Care Centers. The intent of the article is to share with other providers of long term care what works for them to create the best possible environment for people with Alzheimer's disease. Due to the differing needs and abilities of people with Alzheimer's (usually dependent on which stage of the disease they are in), what may work at one facility may not work at another.

10

Ethics

217.   Atkinson, Gary. (1983). "Killing and Letting Die: Hidden Value Assumptions." <u>Social Science Medicine,</u> <u>17</u>(23):1915-1925.

The author discusses a philosophical approach to the complex concept of distinguishing between killing and allowing to die. Case illustrations are used to analyze the moral issues regarding intent, consequences, cause and responsibility. The author considers making a distinction between killing or allowing to die an inadequate and hazardous guide for moral reasoning.

218.   Cassel, Christine K. and Nancy R. Zwiebel. (1990). <u>Public Attitudes about the Use of Chronological Age Criterion for</u> <u>Allocating</u>   <u>Health</u>   <u>Care</u>   <u>Resources:</u>   <u>A</u>   <u>National</u>   <u>Survey</u>. Washington, DC: AARP Andrus Foundation, 45 pages.

This national survey examined the public's perception of age as a basis for health care rationing. Telephone interview data were collected from a representative national sample of 500 adult Americans identified from the national sample frame of the Public Opinion Laboratory of Northern Illinois University. Findings of the study suggest that the American public feels that it is the duty of individual older and younger persons to refuse medical care that would serve only to extend life, especially to extend the lives of persons who are expected to die in a short time. The authors propose that efforts to develop policy in which methods for rationing are delineated must be presented to an informed and experienced public.

219.   Clark, Phillip G. (1991). "Ethical Dimensions of Quality of Life in Aging: Autonomy versus Collectivism in the United States and Canada." The Gerontologist, 31(5):631-639.

The author presents a systematic examination of social ethics as integral to structuring policy and programs that enhance quality of life. The values of autonomy and independence in the United States are compared and contrasted with the Canadian perspective of collectivism and interdependence as dominant values guiding ethical decision-making in the allocation and delivery of health care. The author discusses the importance of combining personal autonomy with an awareness of the larger societal context to form a new gerontological ideology.

220.   Jecker, Nancy S.   (1991).   Aging and Ethics: Philosophical Problems in Gerontology. Clifton, NJ: Humana Press, 394 pages.

A compilation of essays, this book's broad perspective from a multitude of disciplines make it an excellent reference for anyone working with the aged. Issues addressed include the personal experience and meaning of aging, changing family structures, medical decision-making and social responsibility toward our aging society.

221.   Kane, Rosalie A. and Arthur L. Caplan. (1990). Everyday Ethics: Resolving Dilemmas in Nursing Home Life. New York, NY: Springer Publishing Co., 331 pages.

This book offers an unusual and useful approach to sensitizing readers to the ethical dimensions of common occurrences in nursing homes. Following an introduction that establishes a framework, each of 18 chapters begins with a case that embodies a specific ethical issue. Each case is followed by an extensive commentary written by persons who are in a broad sense "ethicists," even though they are drawn from a variety of backgrounds. Also valuable are the "Editors' Questions" at the end of each chapter, which are designed to elicit further discussion. Suggestions for improving the lives of nursing home residents conclude the book.

222.   Kapp, Marshall B. (1992). <u>Ethical Aspects of Health Care for the Elderly: An Annotated Bibliography</u>, Westport, CT: Greenwood Press.

This bibliography cites published material connected by a theme related to "ethical" aspects of geriatric care and spans more than a decade of work from 1980 through the last quarter of 1991. The chapters are organized by topic, with the first devoted to a general overview of sources that deal with ethics, health care, aging and advocacy. Subsequent chapters review autonomy issues, economic factors of health care, caregiving settings, "right to die" issues, functions of ethics committees, problems of medical intervention, advance health care planning, benefits of cadaver use in research, and problems with the use of the elderly as subjects in ongoing medical research.

223.   Kapp, Marshall B. (1991). "Health Care Decision-Making by the Elderly: I Get by with a Little Help from My Family." <u>The Gerontologist</u>, 31(5):619-623.

The author sees the process of health care decision-making as a paradigm of the interdependence between generations. The article explores the ethical and legal considerations in shared decision-making for the mentally capable older adult. When disagreements arise, health care providers, older persons and their families turn to the legal system for answers and clarification of rights and obligations. The legal concept of a "joint medical consent account" is introduced.

224.   Moody, Harry R. (1992). Ethics in an Aging Society. Baltimore MD: Johns Hopkins University Press, 288 pages.

This book reflects on ethical dilemmas as they relate to bioethics, social policy and social ethics. It is divided into three parts. The first addresses ethical issues regarding health care, Alzheimer's disease and rational suicide. The second looks at long term care as it deals with nursing home placement and informed consent. The third part deals with justice between generations as the discussion turns to generational equity and the allocation of scarce health care resources. Ethical questions are discussed in historical, political and theoretical contexts. The author's emphasis on the ideals of autonomy and justice is reflected throughout the book and raises critical questions.

225.   Olson, Ellen et al. (1993). "A Center on Ethics in Long Term Care." The Gerontologist, 33(2):269-274.

Many long term care institutions have created committees to address ethical issues. The Jewish Home and Hospital for the Aged (JHHA) in New York City has taken an innovative approach to ethical issues that provides direct service, case reviews, a research department and an ongoing educational program. These outcomes are achieved through "ethics rounds" where the issues are discussed, and an "ethics consulting team" makes the decisions, along with the family, resident and legal assistance. The problems associated with developing a center on ethics are addressed. Questions of how to ensure the success of such a program are addressed.

226.   Rathbone-McCuan, Eloise and Dorothy R. Fabian (Eds.). (1992). <u>Self-Neglecting Elders: A Clinical Dilemma</u>. New York, NY: Auburn House, 197 pages.

The multifaceted phenomenon of elder self-neglect is presented for clinicians and health care professionals who want to identify, describe and address the problems associated with self-neglect. Discussion of ethical issues incorporates a systems framework and takes into account both psychiatric and biomedical considerations in assessment and intervention. Case examples are presented to show how intervention strategies can be used at different levels of involvement. Chapters on special risks and subgroups address alcoholism, institutional settings and developmental disability. The authors emphasize the need for applied research and experimental programs to deal with this issue.

227.   Waymack, Mark H. and George A. Taylor. (1988). <u>Medical Ethics and the Elderly: A Case Book</u>. Chicago, IL: Pluribus Press, Inc., 256 pages.

Written for the health care professional, this book takes a philosophical approach to ethical concerns of clinical care for the elderly in a modern technological society. A didactic text, it uses cases drawn from real experiences followed by a complete discussion identifying the ethical principles or values involved. Topics include the patient-provider relationship, diagnostic and treatment issues, aspects of locus of care, and the role of finances in health care decision-making. This book is easy to read and an excellent and useful reference for practitioners.

11

Public Policy Issues

Public Policy

228.   Estes, Carroll L. and James H. Swan. (1993). The Long Term Care Crisis: Elders Trapped in the No-Care Zone. Newbury Park, CA: SAGE Publications, 328 pages.

This book analyzes the impacts of recent federal and state health care policy changes, primarily Medicare's prospective payment system for hospitals, on long term care organizations and services, including nursing homes. Supported by extensive research, the central thesis is that communities were and are ill-prepared to accept the responsibility for long term care of the elderly that policy changes have thrust upon them, especially in a period of fiscal constraints. A "no-care zone" has resulted. The final chapters examine arguments for and barriers to needed policy changes. Some knowledge of aging and health care policies is a useful prerequisite to reading this book.

229.   Koff, Theodore H. and Richard W. Park. (1993). Aging Public Policy: Bonding the Generations. Amityville, NY: Baywood Publishing Company, Inc., 341 pages.

The focus of this book is on the formation of public policy for older persons in our society. The authors present a framework for understanding how policy evolves and include a historical overview of aging policy development. The major public policies that affect the older person are presented, along with the processes that led to the establishment of these policies. Finally, the authors comment on the need for future policy changes. The appendices and bibliography provide listings of additional information.

230.   Oriol, William E., compiler (1987). Federal Public Policy on Aging Since 1960: An Annotated Bibliography. Westport, CT: Greenwood Press.

This bibliography covers material concerning federal public policy on aging from 1960 through early 1986. Part one reviews the premises upon which federal aging policy is built. Part two discussed topics which provide an overview of specific programs and issues related to aging. Sub-chapters deal with such wide-ranging concerns as income and retirement policy, health and long term care, housing services, consumer issues, discrimination, education, empowerment, family policy, intergenerational concerns, minorities, research, rural programs, training, and women, and includes an appendix of congressional committees and national organizations. Taking into account the interdisciplinary nature of these topics, the bibliography provides substantial cross-referencing.

231.   Palmore, Erdman B. (1990). Ageism: Negative and Positive. New York, NY: Springer Publishing Company, Inc., 219 pages.

This book defines ageism and suggests useful ways to fight stereotypes about aging, including fostering a better understanding of how future aging developments might be more effectively accommodated through social, governmental and economic policy.

Older Americans Act

232.   Binstock, Robert H. (1991). "From the Great Society to the Aging Society: 25 Years of the Older Americans Act." Generations, 15(3)11-18.

This article chronicles changing attitudes about aging and how the political environment regarding aging programs has changed since the enactment of the Older American Act in 1965.

233.   Gelfand, Donald E. and William Bechill. (1991). "The Evolution of the Older Americans Act: A 25-Year Review of Legislative Changes." Generations, 15(3):19-22.

This article reviews the origins and content of the original OAA, discusses how it has been amended to reflect shifting views of elders, and how the government's role in the well-being of older Americans has changed in concert with these amendments.

Omnibus Budget Reconciliation Act of 1987

234.   Committee on Nursing Home Regulation, Institute of Medicine. (1986). Improving the Quality of Care in Nursing Homes. Washington, DC: National Academy Press, 415 pages.

This report is largely responsible for a policy agenda for reform of federal nursing home regulations, parts of which have been implemented. After examining the concept of quality of care, subsequent chapters examine the issues involved in factors ranging from monitoring nursing home performance and compliance with federal standards to specific recommendations for change and their cost implications. Five appendices, including one on the history of federal nursing home regulations and another on key indicators of quality of care, are useful, as are a glossary of terms and a list of "acronyms and initialisms" in current use.

235.   Gallo, Joseph J. et al. (1991). "Can the New Rules Really Improve Nursing Homes? Omnibus Budget Reconciliation Act (OBRA) Regulations." Patient Care, 25(19):57-62.

The OBRA regulations implemented October 1, 1990, concentrate on resident well-being and patient outcomes. More demanding paperwork and visitations brought on by the new regulations may deter physicians from attending nursing home patients. Some nursing homes have established a closed medical staff, consisting of a small number of physicians who spend a half or a full day caring for several dozen patients within the nursing home. It is argued that physicians on a closed staff may be better acquainted with the necessary procedures and documentation for this type of patient.

236.   Hoyer, Thomas et al. (1990). "Moving Ahead with the Challenge: Making Sense of OBRA." Provider, 16(3):14-20.

This article is composed of four sections. In the first, Thomas Hoyer reviews nursing reform efforts and postulates the composition of successful reform. In the second, Richard Rau discusses quality as it relates to nursing home service delivery. In the third, Barbara Frank focuses on the needs of residents and discusses provider commitment. Finally, Robert Froisness looks at state payment systems that will be necessary to implement the new system and reviews procedural issues.

Financing Long Term Care

237.   Binstock, Robert J. (1992). "Aging, Disability and Long Term Care: The Politics of Common Ground." Generations, 16(2):83-88.

Older persons and younger persons with disabilities have found common ground on policy issues related to long term care but have not yet translated this into unified political action. Problems with the present long term care delivery system are addressed as are Congressional efforts to provide long term care for older persons as well as persons with disabilities. Public perception of a national long term care insurance program by both younger and older Americans is discussed. Since fundamental issues underlying universal health insurance may cause the nation to view long term care as unrelated to age, the author suggests that both the older persons and those who are disabled may be able to unite to achieve increased political representation regarding access issues of long term care.

238.   Geer, Carolyn T. (1991). "The Promises and Pitfalls of Nursing Home Insurance." Forbes, 148:168-170.

The author details some common hazards that consumers should protect against when purchasing long term care policies. Given that almost half of Americans over age 65 will spend some time in a nursing home and that 90% of those who stay more than two years will go bankrupt, insurance that covers nursing home bills warrants consideration. In fact, even under harsh criticism and the high cost of long term care insurance, the industry has grown sevenfold since the mid-1980s. Proposals to set minimum standards for these policies have been offered in Congress but none have been enacted.

239.   Jackson, Mary E. et al. (1992). "Eligibility for Publicly Financed Home Care." American Journal of Public Health, 82(6):853-856.

Proposals for expanding federal coverage of home care include cognitive impairment and activities of daily living as eligibility criteria. Using data from the 1984 National Long Term Care Survey this study concluded that the level of eligibility will have a dramatic effect on the number of older persons who qualify for services and that the number eligible will determine the costs of proposed programs.

240.   Leutz, Walter N. et al. (1991). "Adding Long Term Care to Medicare: The Social HMO Experience." Journal of Aging & Social Policy, 3(4):69-87.

The authors present an overview of the current state-of-the-art of Social Health Maintenance Organizations (SHMO) health delivery demonstration projects in the United States. A discussion of the outcomes and advantages as well as a description of the problems and shortcomings encountered by the model projects are presented. The data sets used were from two of several data sets maintained by the SHMO Consortium (a cooperative research and policy analysis effort of the four demonstration sites and Brandeis University). The data offered in this paper, which focus on feasibility and costs, suggest that it is feasible to define, design and manage an affordable community long term care entitlement.

241.   Liu, Korbin, Pamela Doty and Kenneth Manton. (1990). "Medicaid Spenddown in Nursing Homes." The Gerontologist, 30:7-15.

Under current public policy, individuals are forced to impoverish themselves before getting public assistance through Medicaid for institutional or community-based care. This report presents the findings on nursing home use and spend-down from the 1982 and 1984 National Long Term Care Surveys and the 1985 National Nursing Home Survey. The data demonstrating the number of individuals forced to spend all their assets can be used to evaluate new public policy proposals regarding financing of long term care.

242.   Moses, Stephen A. (1990). "The Fallacy of Impoverishment." The Gerontologist, 30:21-25.

This paper casts doubts upon the common perception that eligibility for Medicaid demands impoverishment. Restrictions on transfer of assets were tightened during the 1980s, but loopholes and lax enforcement have let millions of dollars owed to the states go uncollected because older people transfer their assets to their heirs in order to get Medicaid coverage of nursing home care. The author argues that equitable financing of long term care will require the middle class to choose between public funding of their long term care and preservation of their estates and that people who do not wish to risk encumbering their estates will have to purchase private insurance for catastrophic illnesses.

243.   Quadagno, Jill, Madonna H. Mayer and J. Blake Turner. (1991). "Falling into the Medicaid Gap: The Hidden Long Term Care Dilemma." The Gerontologist, 31:521-526.

This article acknowledges the devastating effects of the spend-down required to qualify for Medicaid, but the researchers are particularly concerned with those whose income is just above the Medicaid cutoff though insufficient to cover the costs of long term care. The "Medicaid Gap" exists primarily in states that exclude individuals receiving institutional long term care from the "medically needy" label required to get public assistance. Because states are only required to provide for the categorically needy (AFDC or SSI recipients) and can set their own income limits, financial assistance can be highly restricted and variable. Furthermore, ineligibility for Medicaid in nursing homes virtually guarantees ineligibility for the alternative home or community-based Medicaid since those limits are even more stringent. For the long run, the only viable solution these authors foresee is devising a national solution to financing long term care.

12

Demographics

244.   Gray, Leonard C., Steven J. Farixh and Michael Dorevitch.   (1992).   "A Population-Based Study of Assessed Applicants to Long Term Nursing Home Care."   Journal of the American Geriatrics Society, 40(6):596-600.

The medical characteristics of applicants to Australian nursing homes were examined in this study.   The data suggest that organic brain disorders were the primary cause necessitating long term care; it was present in 60% of the applicants.   The majority of the applicants (86%) had been ill for more than one year. Dementia was present in 64% of the applicants, and behavioral disturbances were present in 18%.   The authors concluded that efforts to prevent institutionalization should consider the various possible illnesses that could require long term care.

245.   Hurd, Michael D.   (1989).   "The Economic Status of the Elderly."   Science, 244(4905):659-664.

This article reports on the current and projected economic status of older persons in the United States.   The author uses the government poverty rate as a measure of income distribution, suggesting that the substantial number of older persons who are classified as near poor and/or widowed are particularly vulnerable to economic hardship. The definition and conceptualization of economic wealth of older persons is also discussed, taking into consideration that Social Security, Medicare and Medicaid account for 43% of older persons' wealth. The author concludes that in the future, changing dependency ratios, with workers decreasing in relative numbers, will probably lead to the deterioration of the older population's economic status.

246.   Rogers, Andrei, Richard G. Rogers and Alain Belanger. (1990).   "Longer Life but Worse Health? Measurement and Dynamics." The Gerontologist, 30(5):640-649.

This article focuses on the three principal life tables which have been used to calculate active life expectancies: the prevalence rate, the double-decrement and the multi-state models. Data from the 1986 Longitudinal Study of Aging are used to compare the attributes of the three alternative models. The authors contend that all three consider dependency and disability as being irreversible and disregard the impact of recovery on active life expectancy.   A combined model which incorporates both compression of morbidity (delaying the onset of dependency) and expanded recovery, thereby producing an improved active life expectancy, is presented.   Assumptions and calculations underlying each model are presented in graphic form.

247.   Rogers, Richard G., Andrei Rogers and Alain Belanger. (1989).   "Active Life among the Elderly in The United States: Multistate Life-Table Estimates and Population Projections." The Milbank Quarterly, 67(3-4):370-411.

This article presents findings of research to estimate life expectancies for the older adult U.S. population using the data set generated by the 1986 Longitudinal Study of Aging (LSOA) of 5,151 persons aged 70 years and older. Active life measures, mortality rates, multistate life tables and multistate projections were used to calculate active life expectancies. Study findings show that many older adults are living long active lives and that dependency for many is only a temporary or transitional state. Men were found to live a greater proportion of their lives in an active status compared with their female age counterparts. Current trends suggest that as increasing numbers of older persons live to older ages (due to reduced mortality and morbidity), onset of disability tends to increase.

248.   Rogot, Eugene, Paul D. Sorlie and Norman J. Johnson. (1992). "Life Expectancy by Employment Status, Income and Education in the National Longitudinal Mortality Study." Public Health Reports, 107(4):457-460.

This study provides life expectancies for men and women ages 25, 45 and 65, based on data from the National Longitudinal Mortality Study (NLMS) for 1979-85. The study sample consisted of 822,347 noninstitutionalized white persons aged 25-95 years from the NLMS. Findings indicate a direct relationship between increases in income, being employed and higher educational attainment and increases in life expectancy. Life expectancy and income were found to be strongly related; the association between education and life expectancy was not quite as strong.

249.   Seccombe, Karen and Masako Ishii-Kuntz.   (1991). "Perceptions of Problems Associated with Aging: Comparisons among Four Older Age Cohorts."   The Gerontologist, 31(4):527-533.

This research study investigated the perceptions of four older-age cohorts regarding three dimensions of the aging process: the definition of chronological old age, perceived public image of the aged and the major problems/concerns of older persons. Findings indicate that: a) the mean age at which a person is considered old varies among age groups and is extended as the responding individual approaches it; b) the portrayal of older persons by the media is perceived as fair; and c) the youngest age cohort surveyed (ages 55 to 64) perceived the problems most often associated with aging are lack of money, loneliness, inadequate housing, fear of crime and lack of jobs.

Author Index

Note: Numerical entries refer to abstract numbers.

Subject Index

Note: Numerical entries refer to abstract numbers.

About the Compilers

THEODORE H. KOFF, Ed.D., Director of the Arizona Center on Aging and Professor, School of Public Administration and Policy, and the Department of Family and Community Medicine at the University of Arizona, is the author of *Aging Public Policy: Bonding the Generations* (1993), *New Approaches to Health Care for an Aging Population: Developing a Continuum of Chronic Care Services* (1988) and *Long Term Care: An Approach to Serving the Frail Elderly* (1982), among other works.

KRISTINE M. BURSAC, M.P.A., Assistant Director of the Arizona Center on Aging and Director of Project OPEN (Older Person's Emergency Network) and the Crime and the Elderly Study at the University of Arizona, is the coauthor of *More than a Statistic: An Educational Program for Older Adults on Avoiding Criminal Victimization* (1991) and *More than a Statistic: A Training Program on Working with the Elderly for Police Officers* (1991), among other works.

ISBN 0-313-28583-7

90000>

HARDCOVER BAR CODE